# HOPING AND COPING

## HOW MY DARLING LITTLE SON AND I BROKE FREE OF CANCER

# HOPING AND COPING

## HOW MY DARLING LITTLE SON AND I BROKE FREE OF CANCER

By

### Helene Rennervik

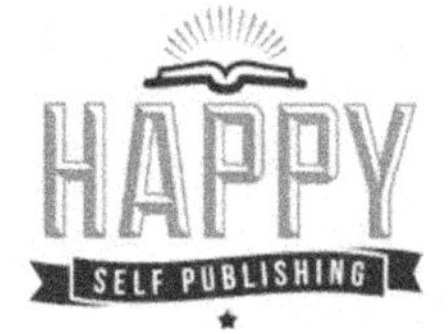

Happy Self Publishing.

# Free Bonus

## FREE PDF TOOL

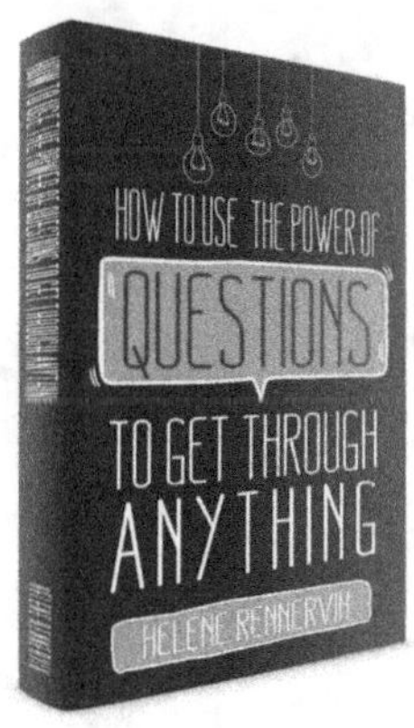


## HOW TO USE
## THE POWER OF QUESTIONS
## TO GET THROUGH ANYTHING

This free PDF is a tool for centering yourself.

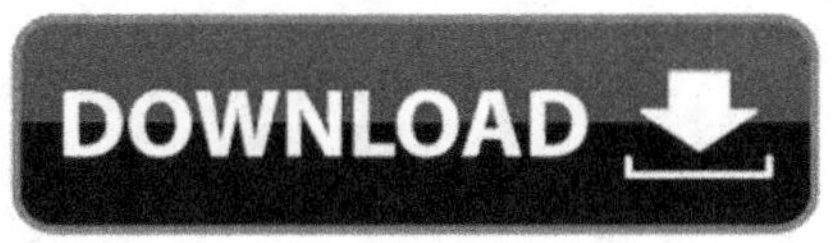


http://helenerennervik.com/book/

# Table of Contents

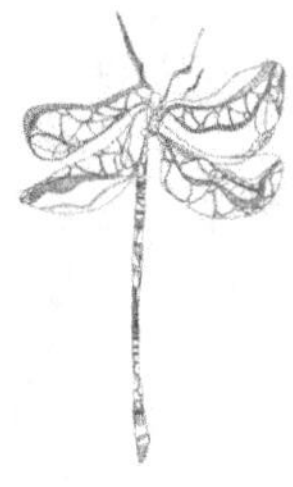

*Love is what we were born with. Fear is what we learned here.*

*– Marianne Williamson*

Dearest,

You Are Not Alone.

You have just found out your child is very sick. Maybe you heard a terrifying diagnosis, or you've gotten lab results that confirm something you (and/or the doctors) suspected.

Sweetheart, I understand. I stood where you are standing. I want to help.

Of course, I cannot make you promises. But, I can be a support when no one else is around in person. I hope I can give you some comfort, some ideas, and resources to see you through the dark nights and to help you find some hope and strength. I called the book "Hoping and Coping" because, for a while, that is all you can do. And, it's enough for now.

I've included exercises for you to use to feel better. I know I can't convince anyone to do them, but I think the book will be more powerful when you do. I've tried to make the story itself strong, for anyone who just doesn't like visualization or meditation or whatever. But, I think you'll get the most out of the book by at least trying the pages that give you something to do. None of them are difficult or take a long time. There might be some that you would like to do with your child. So, if you don't like them for yourself, read through them so that if you are in the middle of a hard day or night with your child, you might remember and use the "tool" to help out the situation.

The world shrinks down so small when your child is sick. It's easy to lose perspective, to grow depressed, to become exhausted. But you don't have to stay there. You can make choices that bring you more "parent-ability" resilience, spirituality, power, and hope.

You can do this. I wish you light on your journey and hope in your heart...

With love,
Helene

# Acknowledgments

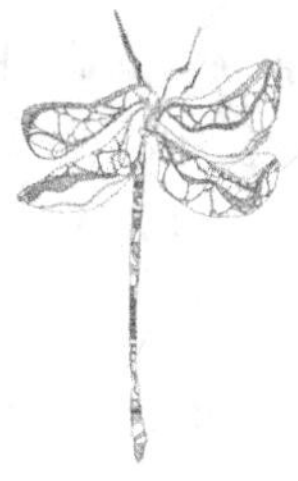

I want to thank my four children, Salina, Nathalie, Laith, and Yousef. I am so proud of, and grateful to, all of them. I thank my family and friends in Dubai, Abu Dhabi, Bahrain, Sweden, and all around the world who supported us, prayed for Yousef, collected money, and came when we needed them. I was so moved by how people responded to us – even people we'd never met. I was amazed by all the gifts, notes, and financial support we received. Thank you, everyone – your kindness means much more than you will ever know.

Because I am grateful for the support we received from the Childhood Cancer Foundation's, a portion of the proceeds from this book will go to support their programming for children who are being treated for cancer, their siblings, and their parents. We were touched by the meals they provided, the excursions, Glädjeverkstan (the clowns), Pysselbyrån (arts& crafts at the wards), and all the little gifts and activities provided to the children and their families. We did not have a big family or network of friends in Sweden. So all the special events and activities sponsored by the Childhood Cancer Foundation helped keep our spirits up. Best of all was the "action day" they had with the police, who brought their dogs to show the children. They came in their cars – which the kids got to ride in with the dogs. Yousef called it, "the best day of my life."

Yousef loved making music and doing arts and crafts. I appreciated the dinners the volunteers made for us since we didn't have many home-cooked meals.

The Childhood Cancer Foundation's support made me feel that I was not alone, but connected to a tribe – maybe not one I would have chosen, but one that made me feel that we belonged to someone. And, we are still a part of this tribe.

Thank you to all of the Q84 doctors and nurses who took care of Yousef, with a special mention to Christoffer Malmström who always looked out for Yousef and who stays still in contact with him, as well as Doctor Otte Brosjö who has made it possible for Yousef to walk again.

I want to thank my coach, Hassan Shaibah, for standing beside me and helping me discover, value, and believe in myself. He helped me set goals and hold myself accountable to achieve them. I would also like to thank Diane Samuels, my book coach, who brought out what was within me to make this book a reality. She knows how to put words to my inner voice.

I have so much appreciation for Akademi Coachstjärnan where I studied for my coaching certification. Here I gained insight and learned the tools to become a great coach.

I look forward to joining Fabian Bolin's War On Cancer platform, with hopes that we can raise awareness and unite more people in the quest for research and a cure for cancer in our lifetime.

# Foreword
# from Fabian Bolin

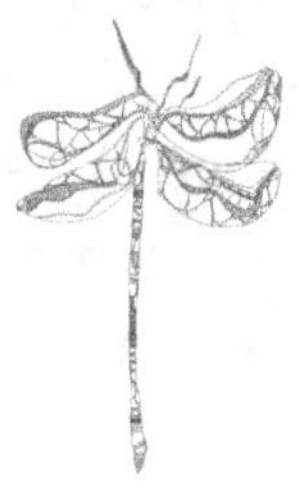

As someone currently going through cancer treatment, I share my journey in a blog because I am very well aware of the power and positive effects of stories. Not only because it helped me immensely to process everything I was going through, but also because my story helped so many others going through the same thing.

When I was diagnosed, the first thing I wanted to find out was what my life would look like for the next two and a half years (the length of my treatment.) I also wanted to know how I could best treat myself alongside the chemotherapy in order to maintain a strong and healthy immune system.

Questions, such as, "what should I eat and not eat?" and "are there any supplements that I can take to boost my health?" were important to me, and they weren't sufficiently answered by my healthcare providers. Hence, I took to the internet to find answers, and they came to me through the people that followed my blog. The knowledge is out there, and thanks to wonderful people like Helene, who has real and genuine experience from a parenting perspective, others can learn.

What I find most captivating about Helene is her energy. From the moment I met her I could sense her passion and drive to help parents in similar situations. I could see it in her eyes that she's a doer and I have no doubt that her work will help thousands of people, if not millions.

Fabian Bolin is the CEO and co-founder of WarOnCancer.com, an empowering social platform for everyone affected by cancer - patients, survivors, and their loved ones. The focus lies on mental health and recovery through storytelling, connection, and financial support. WarOnCancer.com aims to play an integral part in modernizing mental healthcare and is already collaborating with several hospitals in order to incorporate the service as a tool for healthcare professionals. Fabian is currently undergoing treatment for acute lymphoblastic leukemia and has been brought into the management team for the Department of Hematology, Oncology and Endocrine tumors at Uppsala University Hospital.

After being diagnosed with leukemia in 2015 at 28 years of age, Fabian began documenting his cancer battle on a blog, which quickly gained global attention. His first post, shared over 13,000 times on Facebook, has led to over 100,000 messages, emails, and letters of support to date. He later won the award "Journalist of the Year 2015" for his blog by CancerRehabFonden.

By recognizing the power and potential of storytelling, and combining it with a strong urge to empower others affected, the idea of #WarOnCancer was born. A movement to unite the world.

# Dedication

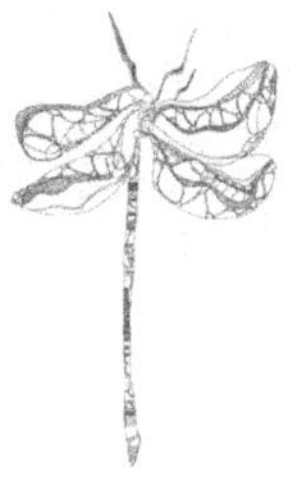

This book is dedicated to my son Yousef, who I love beyond words, and to all the children and parents who must take this cancer journey. I pray for your courage and hope.

# Introduction

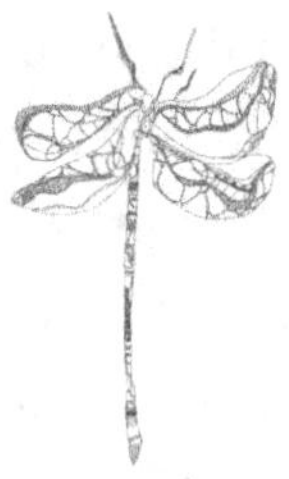

Today, as I sit down to write, it is gray and chilly - 3.1° in Stockholm. We are expecting snow in the next few days. I am a world away from my old life in Dubai, my home for over 25 years, where I raised my children and worked as a personal trainer. Right now, Dubai is almost 26° and sunny. Had our life not been altered so dramatically, today, I might be planning an afternoon with my daughter Salina and Aya my grand-daughter at the Dubai Mall or the beach. As it is, I have to be satisfied with speaking with them through Skype, WhatsApp, and Instagram.

Had things been different, my youngest child would be at his football (soccer) practice, and innocently enjoying his comfortable life with his family and friends. Maybe we would stop off at Salina's house on our way home for the evening, or we'd be planning to go out to one of the many great restaurants at the Walk or Al Wasl Square.

As it is, we don't live near our family or Yousef's familiar school and friends anymore. We have a new home in the country where I was born. We are only 12 minutes away from the hospital where we spend so much time. The life we have today would have been unimaginable even two years ago.

We live overlooking a big field with a flood-lit football court. Yousef doesn't go there. I have seen him watch some games from our living room window. He misses being able to play. We live on the outskirts of Stockholm – on the north side. It's not my favorite place to live, but I was very fortunate to get a contract on an apartment. I would have liked to live in the center of Stockholm in an old refurbished building, but, the prices were far too high, and not knowing what will happen with Yousef, I couldn't use all my savings to invest in an apartment. Maybe in the future, we'll see. I would like Yousef to grow up in a nice neighborhood where he feels safe. Yousef would prefer a house in the countryside where he could have the German Shepherd he wants so badly by his side.

I am new here in my own country. Except for Yousef, I'm separated from my kids. Salina, my eldest, is in Dubai with her husband, Liam, and their little daughter, Aya. Salina is a very feeling person. She cares deeply about others and wants to make a difference. Salina is a play therapist, working with children. She wants them to be able to express themselves, so they can heal, using more than words alone. My second daughter, Nathalie, finished at the London College of Fashion in May 2015. She is a designer focusing on sustainable, cutting-edge fashion. Both she and her brother, Laith, have a desire to do the right thing for the earth, to care for it, to make a difference in the world. Laith has recently started at Queen Mary University, in London. He is studying sustainable energy engineering. Samer Yousef's father is also in Dubai.

I am building my coaching business, scheduling regular sessions via Skype and in person while networking to get myself out there: meeting different people to get my business up and running. It was so much easier in the United Arab Emirates, (UAE) where I knew loads of people and where people knew me.

I am writing now while I have a few moments because soon, I will have to pick Yousef up from school and get him to the Astrid Lindgren's Hospital for his physiotherapy appointment. After that, we need to go to Team Olmed and meet Johannes, who is an Orthopedic Engineer. He will check the inlays in Yousef's shoes, which compensate for the fact that his left leg is shorter than the right. Yousef likes to go to these appointments because they have a machine that makes yummy hot chocolate.

Right now, a treatment my son needs is being held up by a medical supply company for reasons no one understands. Yousef grows. The machine that lengthens his leg by tiny increments, and which gives him a chance to develop more normally, is caught up in some international bureaucracy for the last four months and hasn't been delivered to the hospital. As I watch Yousef adapt to his shortened leg, I wonder where in the world this machine is, and how the children who need it can be treated so coldly. Medical companies change hands, money is made, children wait, and the rest of the world seems to go on as usual.

But, our lives will go on as well. I have the good fortune to look back now, knowing Yousef is cancer-free. I know we still have challenges ahead as he will have check-ups and follow-ups and will be watched closely for many years yet. But, today, I am grateful.

I want to help parents who are where I was only a few short years ago by sharing my story. You might see bits of your experience in mine, but of course, every family, treatment, and child is so different. What is terrible is the sameness: the cancer that brings us together at this moment.

# Your Feelings

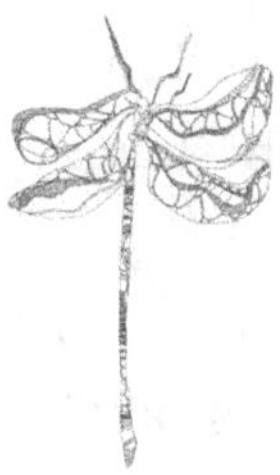

---

*"Bad news is that you can control nothing but your thoughts. Good news is that with your thoughts you can control everything else."*

*–Debasish Mridha*

---

How do we let in devastating news without being crushed or immobilized? How do we take that next unimaginable and inevitable step forward toward God knows what? How do we find peace of mind when there is no peace in us?

Even in that "oh my God" state, you can acknowledge that you can get a hold of your mind. When events are beyond our control, the one thing we do have is our conscious choices and our powerful questions, such as: what do I do now with this situation?

If you don't accept this idea, think about a time when one crisis followed immediately after another. All of a sudden, the first thing faded, and the other became HUGE.

I have a friend who says, "Never say it can't get worse because it always can!" But, I say it can always get better.

*Let me give you an example. We were having a terrible day. I couldn't imagine anything worse, and I couldn't detach my thoughts and feelings from it. I stayed in the "worry about it" stage for hours. Then, something shocking happened. Now my thoughts and feelings were focused on something entirely different. Where did the old feelings go? Why did those huge, obsessive feelings now seem so insignificant?*

**When you start to pay attention, you will see your feelings come up and fade away like waves on the beach. Up they come and almost swamp you. Then, they recede around your feet. How might you let them rise and fall away without taking you out to sea?**

Before you say, "I can't do that!" consider this: it's just your mind telling you a story. It can easily change from "this is terrible" to "OK, this will be a challenge that we can get through and be better for at the end."

**What are you telling yourself right now?**

How might something better be true? What might be some alternative thought, one that will give you hope? Even if it is outrageous, ask, "what if…?"

# CHAPTER ONE

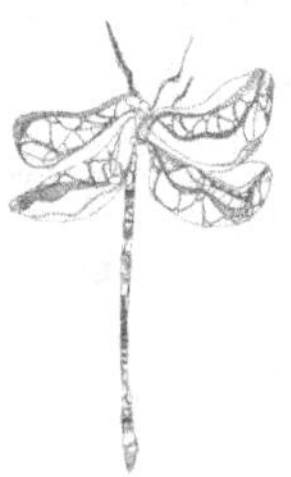

# Not Like Any Other Day

---

*"It's strange how the worst day of your life often starts just like any other. You might even complain very quietly to yourself about its ordinariness. You might wish for something more interesting to happen, something to back off your routine, and just when you think you can't bear the monotony any longer, something comes along that shatters your life to such degree, you wish with every cell in your body that your day hadn't become so unordinary."*

*–Joanna Cannon*

---

February 1, 2015 was a Sunday, the first day of the week in Dubai. As always, I was the first one up. I moved around quietly so I wouldn't wake Samer while I fixed my hair and make-up and got dressed in my gym clothes. It was a strength training day for my first client in Jumeirah. Before I got to work though, I had my nine-year-old son to get up and ready. I crept into Yousef's room and pulled the curtains aside. I climbed up into his bunk bed and kissed him, never imagining it would be the last time I would ever do this.

"Good morning, Yousef! Time to get up!" I said.

He is so cute in the morning when he is still sleepy. He didn't fuss much, but got up and dressed in his uniform of a white and purple shirt with navy blue shorts and socks.

In the kitchen, I made my Swedish coffee "to go," enjoying its amazing smell. While I waited for Yousef, I drank some lemon water and ate a banana, thinking how lucky I was that my first client always made me a sandwich to take with me after I trained with her.

Yousef had his cereal, and I looked out my living room window. There still wasn't too much traffic on the extremely busy Sheikh Zayed Road. Dubai is one of the world's most cosmopolitan cities. It is changing fast, building and growing, getting more congested all the time. It is a wonderful location, near the desert and also the beach. Yousef calls it "hot like an oven with buildings everywhere you go." In Dubai, you can find every designer store, luxury brand, international restaurant, and a mingling of people from all over the world, including expats like me. We lived between two metro stops, and I watched the train going by. Now that scene is captured in my mind, a snapshot of my former life.

Before eight o'clock, I'd dropped Yousef off at school and was walking through my client's beautiful garden of fragrant flowers, palm and orange trees on my way to her elegant house. As always, she came down the stairs into her private gym at 8:00 on the dot, smiling. I felt lucky to work with this lovely and gracious woman. This was my life, so easy and pleasant.

After our session, I stopped at the supermarket before going home where Samer helped me make cosa, Yousef's favorite dish. Samer scooped out the center of the small zucchini, and I stuffed it with minced meat and rice. I love cooking, and we all enjoy eating healthy food, especially Lebanese, my children's favorite. I used to make it all the time, but now these little routines have become just precious memories.

Yousef loves football, and he played after school two or three days a week. I usually picked him up after 2.30 on Sunday but on this day our routine was interrupted by a call.

"Helene! It's Suzy! You've got to come down to the school right away! Yousef hurt his leg – it might be broken."

"What happened?" I asked, alarm bells going off in my head.

"He was running, and all of a sudden, he fell and started screaming," she said.

I tried to take this in. Wasn't it just a fall? It happens all the time in soccer.

"The nurse told him not to move his leg. Should we call the ambulance?" Suzy asked.

"Let me call his dad," I said.

Samer was out with the car, and he picked up the phone immediately. Fortunately, he was close by, so he rushed over to the school ahead of me. I ran downstairs and tried to hail a taxi. How is it when you urgently need something, it is so much harder to get a hold of? Maybe it just seems that way.

I finally got into a taxi and told the driver to get me to Rashid Hospital as fast as he could. I couldn't believe it when he took a wrong turn and went in the opposite direction. Anxious and frustrated, I eventually arrived at the hospital to find Yousef sitting in a wheelchair, looking very lost and worried.

They set Yousef's leg in a cast and told us he'd be on crutches and out of school for six weeks. I took a picture of Yousef looking very dejected – he was in pain, and sad that he wouldn't be playing football for who knew how long. In a picture from the following day, he looks better: in a cast with his leg sticking straight out, but cheered up by the Nerf gun that his big brother, Laith, brought him.

My biggest concern was contacting his teachers about picking up homework and speaking to Lynn, the school nurse. I was thinking about all the classes he'd miss and wondering how I would wash him with the cast on. I was preoccupied with all the details of a kid with a broken leg. A school holiday was coming up, so while he'd miss some school, it wouldn't be quite so bad. As for Yousef, it wasn't long before he was hopping around on his crutches, and we were able to take him out a little bit.

About three weeks later, feeling very cooped up and ready to get back to school, Yousef had his friend Mo over to play. Suddenly, I heard Yousef screaming. I ran into his room to find him lying on the floor. I thought they had been jumping around or something, but Mo said Yousef had only tripped over his crutches. Mo stood there horrified, watching Yousef screaming on the floor. His pain and panic seemed over the top. I thought he was mostly scared since it wasn't a big fall. I tried to get him to stop crying, and he calmed down a little, although he was still in pain. After Mo went home, I called a friend who told me about a homeopathic medicine for pain, which we had the pharmacy deliver. I gave to Yousef, but it didn't work very well. I couldn't understand his strong reaction to falling. He couldn't have broken his leg again – who has ever heard of that? To break a leg that's already in a cast?

Because he was in pain all night, we took him to the hospital the next morning where his leg was x-rayed. Sure enough, the ER doctor told us it had broken again. Both Samer and I could see something was off with the x-ray. It didn't look like a clean break – something was there, but of course we had no idea what we were looking at. What did we know? That afternoon I was surprised when a different doctor called. He said he'd been looking over the x-ray and noticed something the doctor from the ER had missed.

Assuring us there was probably nothing to worry about, he recommended I bring Yousef back to the hospital to have his leg checked. By this time, Samer had gone out of town, but when I called and told him what the doctor said, he had a family friend come with us to the ER where we checked Yousef into the hospital. On Monday, he had blood tests and a CT scan of his leg. He stayed in the hospital overnight.

On Tuesday morning, our lives changed forever. I will never forget standing alone in a hallway in Rashid Hospital listening to doctors tell me that my son had cancer. They suspected it was Ewing's sarcoma.

"What is that?" I asked.

"Cancer of the bone."

Were these men actually telling me my son had bone cancer?

Two of the doctors left, and one stayed and kept talking. He said they could do a biopsy at another hospital in Dubai. I was shocked to hear what he advised next.

"Go back to your country," he said.

I am Swedish, but I've lived in Dubai for over 25 years. What was he talking about? Dubai was my home.

"Is that because you're afraid it will spread?" I asked.

He explained that this was a very rare type of cancer and required a special operation.

"They don't have specialists here for children's cancer," he said.

"Do you have children?" I asked. He said yes.

"Where would you take your child?"

"Germany," he said.

Was I hearing right? Was he telling me to leave my home? And go where? To Sweden or Germany? My thoughts were swirling around the idea of a malignant tumor in Yousef's leg. I wanted to know, if it was cancer, what stage? Was it spreading? I had

so many questions, and such turmoil in my head --
and my child was in another room with no idea what
was going on. How would I tell him?

As thoughts came and went, the doctor's voice
faded. Actually, everything around me sounded
muffled. I felt completely removed from the world,
detached, as if I were watching from a distance.
Eventually, I turned away from the doctor, focusing
on a door at the end of the long corridor. I walked
down that endless hallway, noticing out of the corner
of my eye that the walls were moving past me.
Finally, I pushed open the door at the end of the hall
and went down the stairs in a trance. Nothing felt
real.

Yousef's father was still away, at an exhibition in
Doha, Qatar. He'd been out of work for a while and
looking for a job was a high priority. I was all alone,
and soon I'd have to talk to my son. I realized hadn't
written anything down, not a single note about what
the doctors had said, and I was confused about the
details.

I called Samer, still in a daze. He had so many
questions, and I just couldn't answer them. I heard
the fear and frustration in his voice. But, I wondered
what it mattered to have all that information – what
would we do with it all? My feeling was that no
matter what, we were going to have to find a doctor
we trusted and put our faith in him or her. In spite of

my own questions, a part of me had decided that already.

Throughout our ordeal, I felt so much pressure to do exactly what the doctors demanded. It was intense to take in so much information. I was often left with questions and sometimes, misunderstanding. I wasn't even sure what questions to ask because medical opinions were given to me as facts, with no alternatives. I often had a hard time remembering conversations that had just happened a few hours before, or even who was in the room with me then!

I'd try to remember to bring a notepad and jot down what the doctor said, but I often forgot. It was good when I had someone go with me because then we could re-create the conversation afterward.

I learned not to be afraid to ask a doctor to repeat himself. I believe they are the expert, but not the "authority." Sometimes they could be intimidating, but I decided they are there to help me understand and make the right decisions for my child.

That first day, I was completely unprepared. I had no paper, no pen. I had no idea what news I would hear, and I was in such a state of shock, I just couldn't help Samer with his questions.

Samer hung up and must have called his whole family in Lebanon right away, because immediately, everyone was calling their doctors and looking into what Ewing's sarcoma was. Soon all their advice and search results would come at us fast and furious. I know they were trying to help, but it only made us more anxious.

After that, word spread fast among our friends and acquaintances. All over the world, people looked into what Yousef had. At the same time, the opinions started: go to Italy, go to Beirut, go to the United States, go straight to Sweden.

Somehow, I made it down the corridor to Yousef's room. He was lying in bed. I tried to keep myself from crying so I wouldn't frighten him.

"I'm going downstairs to the coffee shop. Would you like something?" I asked.

"No," he said.

I walked out of the room, still in a trance, with that same thought playing in a loop over and over: your son has cancer.

I got in line for coffee; I was completely numb. I called my daughter, Salina. Although she wouldn't normally pick up the phone when she was at work, this time she did.

"The doctors just came and talked to me. They told me that Yousef has cancer. They think it's Ewing's sarcoma," I told her. Salina told me later how strange my voice sounded.

On the other end of the phone, I heard her sharp gasp. Hot tears started streaming down my face. Like a robot, I moved forward in the line to the counter, tears pouring down as I ordered a latte. I guess the people working there thought I was crazy. Or maybe they are used to it?

Salina promised we would talk to Yousef together. In the UAE, family comes first, so as soon as she told her employer what had happened, they let her leave work to come and be with us.

As Yousef's mother, I was so close to it, so emotionally involved, that Salina really took hold of the situation when I needed the support. She was like an extra mother to Yousef. Ever since she was small, she has always carried so much for her sister and brothers. Salina said that she realized right away that her role would be to support me so that I could support Yousef. I couldn't have done it without her.

"What shall I tell him? How shall I tell him he's got cancer? What's the best way to tell a child?" I asked her. I had so many questions.

"Let me call Lara in the UK," she said. Lara was her clinical supervisor and a play therapist as well. "Let's see what she advises is the best way."

"What about Nathalie and Laith?" I ask.

"Don't worry, Mamma, I'll tell them," Salina said.

I sat down outside the entrance of the coffee shop for what must have been 30 or 40 minutes, tears flowing. People were coming and going past me, but I didn't care. By the time I walked back upstairs and got to Yousef's room, I had gotten myself together.

"Where did you go for so long, Mamma?" Yousef asked.

"Oh, it took some time to get the coffee," I said.

He was sitting in bed playing, my darling son. Thoughts were running wild in my mind. Is he going to die? I wondered. What can I do for him? How would I tell him this terrible news?

Now I think about how long I was away from him, and I wonder what he must have been thinking. Does it make me a bad mother? At the time, it wasn't a conscious decision to stay away, but I was putting one foot in front of the other, the best I could. It wasn't perfect, but it was good enough.

Later that afternoon, Yousef was scheduled for an MRI. This was a big deal for him.

"No!" he said, "I am not going in there!"

I wish someone had explained why he needed the MRI, how it would work, what he could expect. But, no one did, and I didn't know enough to tell him myself. Coming right after the shock of breaking his leg for the second time, and now being hospitalized, it was a lot for a nine-year-old boy to process.

During the test, the noises of the machine terrified him. This traumatic experience at the very beginning of our cancer journey made every test and procedure that much harder for him. Fear was embedded, and it was hard to let it go. Eventually, he'd have to go under anesthesia for most of his scans. If there had been a way to ease him into that first MRI experience, it would have helped us later. It taught me something about how to talk to my son – and how important it would be to help him control his fear and anxiety as we went along.

I was going through my own anxiety, too. There was very little time to process my emotions, which would have helped me help *him*. I couldn't wait to talk to my other children and my friends, even though, I wasn't sure what I'd say. I hoped someone would have just the right contact or the right advice to guide me. Soon, Samer would be home, and we could talk about what would be best for Yousef.

## Accepting What Is

No matter how you hear the news, whether you suspected something was wrong or not, whether you are alone or with someone else, hearing the diagnosis for the first time will be a shock. And now, for a while, your life will be disrupted in ways you could never have expected.

**What is the best possible thing now?**

Your partner/spouse will have different communication styles, questions, reactions, fears, feelings, and beliefs than you do.

**What is the gift in these differences between you?**

You will get a barrage of information from well-meaning others.

**What if all this research they are doing is making them feel better? What if it isn't about you at all? Can you let that be?**

Like Yousef, your child might have a hard time with bad news, tests, and procedures. One friend I have tells her 7-year-old son he's going to have a blood test. First, he freaks out. Then, he goes to his room for a while, and later, comes downstairs, completely ready to handle the test.

What if your child could tell you what is best for them? What if you weren't afraid to ask him/her but trusted the deep wisdom inside them?

## My Notes

# CHAPTER TWO

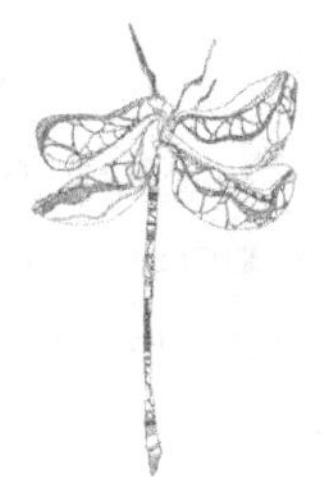

# Will I Die?

---



*"When we face death, really face it, we realize that only love matters."*

*- Marty Rubin*

---

Later that afternoon, Salina and I sat down with Yousef. He knew he had more than just a broken bone, since here he was, back in the hospital for more tests.

"We have to tell you something big. We heard back about the tests you had," Salina said. She paused and gauged Yousef's reaction.

"They see something on your femur." She pointed to his leg. "They think it is cancer in your bone. That's why it broke three weeks ago, and again, this time."

Salina waited, watching Yousef. Her tone was very reassuring; her words were child-friendly. She made a point to keep each sentence short. Later, she explained she had gone into her professional mode: using "therapeutic pauses," just the way she would with her young play-therapy clients.

Salina assuring him anyone would be surprised to hear this kind of news. Pacing herself so she wouldn't overwhelm him with details, she mentioned other people in our family who'd gotten cancer.

"You know Uncle Omar had cancer, and he had special treatment and got well. Remember, it was the same with Auntie Jill and Auntie Liselotte."

We left out people in our family who had died from cancer. Salina told Yousef that the doctors would have to do a biopsy.

"The doctors take a piece of the bone to look at in the lab. Then, they'll know what type of cancer you have and what the best treatment for you will be."

Salina knew he would be scared to hear all this. The whole time, Yousef was mostly worried about whether things would hurt. When it was an injection, we'd have to tell him honestly that yes, it might hurt. If he was just scheduled for an x-ray, we could tell him it would be painless and quick. He asked about the biopsy.

"You'll be sleeping. You won't feel it," Salina said.

In fact, when he woke up from the biopsy he was in terrible pain, with a pump so he could give himself a dose of morphine when he needed it.

We both told Yousef that we would do everything we could for him – that everyone, friends, family, doctors, and nurses all would do the same. Yousef just stared at us. I wondered what I could do to make it easier for him. Salina asked him if he had any questions.

"Will I die?" Yousef asked. Children can be so blunt!

"God willing, they will have a treatment. Everyone is trying to find the best way for you to get well," she said. "We're also checking to see if it would be better for you to go to another country."

"I don't want to hear any more," Yousef said.

"OK. If you think of anything – anything at all – you can ask us later, anytime," Salina said.

The tension in my body and on my face must have been very obvious. Salina took me aside to remind me that Yousef could pick up on my feelings.

"Children are more intuitive than we give them credit for," she said. "He senses your stress; he can see the worry on your face. If you haven't processed information before you talk to him, you might add even more anxiety to whatever he feels."

From then on, I became super-aware of that. Whenever I could, I took a moment for myself to breathe and look around. I allowed myself to become aware of my surroundings, and I made a practice of looking for some small thing to appreciate. Focusing on that one beautiful color or lovely scene kept me in the moment and helped me stay centered. Then I could remind myself there is always enough time to say it slowly, and in the right way.

Throughout the whole process, I learned to notice when Yousef had enough information. He would become like a snail or a roly-poly curling in on himself. You could see it in his face when he had shut down. Even though he might be nodding at us as if he were listening, his eyes would wander, or he might look as if he was going to cry. We became sensitive to those signs, and we'd stop talking. I realized that explanations can always be filled in for him later if he wanted to know.

I felt so much pressure in the beginning. I had to gather information. I had to hurry up and make decisions. I only had a limited time with the doctors to ask all my questions. I worried I would forget some, and later, it would be too late to ask. Some doctors were very patient with us and took their time. Others made us feel even more nervous because they didn't have a very good bedside manner, or weren't great with children. With some of them, we overlooked arrogance or impatience because of their experience, confidence, and skill.

I was juggling what Yousef should hear and what I needed to know. As I was trying to figure out how to tell Yousef things, Salina helped me realize I was going through my own trauma about my child's illness. It's a lot for a parent. Salina could see when I was reacting because I was flustered or still in shock myself. She told me to process information myself first, but honestly, in the beginning, when things were being thrown at me so fast, it was hard not to react emotionally.

"How do I comfort him while I'm handing him over to these scary things at the same time?" I asked.

"Reassure him!" Salina said. "Even if that's all you can do. Tell him you'll be there, that he'll never be alone. That's good enough."

All of us believed it was best to be completely honest with Yousef. We always told him the truth, even if it was difficult. Not every family will decide to do it this way. For example, when Yousef asked if he would die, we honestly said we didn't know.

"Yousef, it's not only kids who have cancer. Nobody knows when their time will come," I said.

Yousef was nine, and with a younger child we might have done something different, but we decided as long as we went slow and watched his reactions, we'd tell him the plain truth. Salina said we had to follow our gut instinct. If we thought he'd reached his limit for the day, we gave him something else to focus on, a game or toy or TV show. If it'd been a hard day of testing or treatment, we wouldn't put more pressure on him by giving him information. We would just let him be.

Whenever we could, we let him lead the conversation. Sometimes there were things he needed to know right then – we didn't want to surprise him with procedures or tests. We learned to be very sensitive to signs that said, "I'm done!" *without* Yousef having to say it. If I wasn't sure, I'd say something like "Maybe you don't feel like talking about it now, that's OK, we can later," or, "You can tell me when to stop."

Salina reminded me that if it seemed like he was worried about something, it was okay to ask, "I wonder if you are feeling worried?" Usually, he didn't have to say a word because I could see it on his face, and it broke my heart because there was never enough reassurance to make the worry go away.

Yousef went back and forth between shutting down and asking questions. Salina told me that just as "I wonder..." is a good sentence starter, "I don't know," is a perfectly fine (and honest) sentence too.

It turned out there was so much I just didn't know. It was a relief to let that be, for Yousef, and for me.

### How to Speak to Your Child

Let them ask.

Let them lead the way.

Only answer what they are asking. Unless they want details, don't add any.

If you don't know the answer, be honest: "I don't know. Let's ask the doctor."

If you are worried, go take some time to yourself so you can be calm when you talk. You can say, "I want to talk to you about that. Let me give you a hug, and may I have just a minute first, so I can answer you in the best way?"

If you have news they won't like to hear, tell the child it is OK for them to be in charge of what they hear: "Tell me when you've had enough." "Tell me when you want me to stop."

"You can always ask me questions. If I don't know, we can ask the doctor or the nurse."

"You can always ask me later."

"I wonder how you are feeling?"

"I wonder if there is anything you want to know?"

"What would make you feel better right now?"

"No matter when you want to talk, it's OK."

"There are no topics that are off-limits, even scary things."

"It's OK if you don't want to talk about it."

"It's OK if you don't want to know the details."

"Tell me when you've heard enough."

"It's OK to cry."

"What do you need right now to feel a bit better?"

## My Notes

# CHAPTER THREE

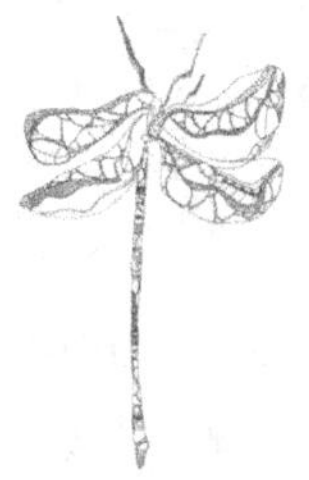

# Dr. Who?

---

*"The pain you feel today is the strength you feel tomorrow. For every challenge encountered, there is opportunity for growth."*

*— Unknown*

---

My first instinct was to support Yousef with positivity, but I might have gone a little over the top! That night, right after the (unconfirmed) diagnosis, Yousef had to stay in the hospital. I asked Salina to call our family and friends and tell them they could come visit Yousef. I told them to bring a smile and happiness only. I basically asked them not to show their fear or worry but to support Yousef by being positive.

Many of our friends and relatives came that evening. We brought food and had a party in his room. Yousef got so much attention, so many toys and gifts, it was a happy night for him, which is what I wanted. But now I think he was spoiled by all the presents and all the attention, maybe confused too, having a party after the bad news of earlier that day. He had no idea what was coming. I wonder if I did the right thing – pumping him up only to have him crash to earth with what came next. He wasn't prepared, but how could I prepare a 9-year-old to leave his friends and family and face cancer treatment in a foreign country? How could I even get him to grasp it all? Looking back, I see how completely clueless we all were.

That night I went home and finally slept. It is normal to be in a kind of trance when something so shocking happens. You don't sleep or eat right; you don't function well. You just do what you have to do: go back and forth to the hospital. Order food. Handle the small things.

Then, there are the big decisions to be made as well. We were gathering up the medical reports and sending copies to doctors outside the country to find the best treatment we could. We had no idea what hospital – or even what country! -- would be the best for Yousef, and many people tried to be helpful and give their advice. It was overwhelming, but in the end, only Samer and I could decide what would be best for Yousef. We both favor natural methods of healing, but hearing how urgent Yousef's condition was, I decided to trust the doctors.

My younger daughter Nathalie was surprised I was even considering chemo, but Salina said, "Do what's best for Yousef."

I spoke to my friend Jill (who is also Salina's mother-in-law and a cancer survivor herself). She had some very useful contacts in Dubai and elsewhere, and both she and her husband had been treated for cancer in Germany. She is a very strong person, someone I relied on a lot, so I asked her to help. Jill had a contact in Abu Dhabi, a man who expedites medical treatment abroad for those who need it. He started locating doctors for Yousef right away. He knew we had to keep costs down, as we would be paying for treatment ourselves.

We were in an unusual situation because we were only residents of Dubai. Had we been citizens, the government or possibly even a wealthy private patron would have helped us pay for medical care. There is so much wealth there, it wouldn't be unusual, especially when a child is involved. On the other hand, if we were residents of the European Union, Yousef could have been treated anywhere in Europe. As a non-resident, he was not covered.

I tried to keep the financial aspect in perspective, but I admit it was in my mind as we tried to find the right treatment for Yousef's rare cancer. We wanted the best for him, but we did not have the funds to pay for it. Samer had been out of work for quite some time, and our savings would not cover the hundreds of thousands of Euros medical care would cost.

Yes, we would need to come up with a great deal of money, but I decided I would just have to trust that it would come from somewhere. I had to trust that the right care would come, first.

I was overwhelmed by everything we found on the internet. Then, add to that, the number of people who were searching, too! The internet is wonderful, but I wouldn't go there for information right away, even though that seems to be everyone's first instinct.

I think it's overwhelming at a point when your brain is already overloaded with information from the doctors, and you're probably in a state of shock. I know to go to reputable sites, such as hospitals, cancer centers, and cancer societies, but the stories of what other parents have been through still drew my attention, and I had to tell myself to avoid them.

I was not that big a Facebook user, but for many people, social media is a lifeline and even a way of life! Facebook is another place where friends can focus on the worst things and put terrible stories and cases and things they "heard" in one's mind. But it's OK to just tell them not to. I wanted to tell people, only "likes" friends! Thank you!" Otherwise, I ran the risk of wondering "what if" all those terrible things happen to my child!

One woman I know asked one of her friends to handle the communication for her. Every day they'd talk, and then the friend would post on Facebook. She never reported back what any of the replies were. Almost all the comments were supportive, and only if there was something like an offer of <u>useful</u> help, did she break the rule and tell us.

I think we have to take charge of how we use social media and ignore posts, emails, texts, and whatever overwhelms us. I realized I didn't have to tell everyone everything or even answer every email. I decided to handle it however, and worry about offending people later!

I wanted to start a blog and post all the developments regularly. I thought it would be good for me, and it would let our loved ones know what was happening. But, I didn't know how involved everything would be – and what could happen that would take all my attention. I gave up the idea pretty fast, though I did record notes in my phone when I could, and I took a lot of pictures, so I could remember to write things down later. The pictures have helped me to reconstruct the story for this book.

The doctors told us that Yousef needed to have a biopsy right away so they could see for sure the type of cancer he had, whether it had spread, and what stage it was at. They kept telling us that there was no time to wait, and we would have to decide right then. It was so much pressure. I understand the importance of going fast, but now, looking back, I see how there is a line you cross with cancer treatment, and then there is no going back. It felt like we had stepped onto a treadmill and could not get off.

We knew for sure we couldn't stay in Dubai – there just weren't sufficient cancer services for children there. I thought about going back to Sweden, but I didn't know the process. All this time, we had people making calls and offering suggestions. I trusted Jill, so I followed her recommendations instinctively. So much pressure was building up in my head that when Jill called to tell me a doctor was willing to see us, I didn't question anything; I just felt an incredible weight lift from my shoulders. I felt hope: soon Yousef would be getting treated. Now, a doctor who actually knows about children's cancer would accept my son as his patient. Even as I write this, many months later, I feel the same chills run through my body, because with that "yes," there was hope.

The problem was, I wasn't processing everything quite right. Once Jill mentioned Heidelberg, and I started doing research, I got it into my head that's where we would be going: to Heidelberg University Hospital, to see a specialist named Dr. Ho. This wasn't the case at all! Jill's contact had found a government hospital in Karlsruhe, Germany where a Dr. Schmittenbecher was willing to see Yousef right away. As anxious as we were to get answers and start some sort of treatment, we had no choice but to put him off, so we could arrange travel and take care of things at home. He agreed to see us that Monday.

I guess I assumed Dr. Schmittenbecher was an associate of Dr. Ho. I had no idea where Karlsruhe was; I thought it must be in or near Heidelberg. I have to laugh now at how naïve both Samer and I were. Who gets on a plane without knowing where they're going? How do you even read the departures board if you don't know the destination? We still didn't realize, even when the plane landed and we were met by a stranger who proceeded to drive us many miles, in the middle of the night to the town of Karlsruhe. At home, I'd told everyone about this great doctor and hospital in *Heidelberg.*

"It's the best, the top of the top, world-class treatment!" I said, wanting to give Yousef faith and hope.

"You're going to this amazing hospital! You are such a lucky boy, because not all children get to see this wonderful doctor!"

In a text to Suzie, who'd called me when Yousef broke his leg, I wrote,

*"Yesterday, the best possible doctor for Yousef's case agreed to treat him! He is in Germany, and we will travel on Sunday. I've asked everyone to stay calm and happy. All I ask is that Yousef feels secure, safe, and happy. He is only a little boy, so it's a lot for him to go through. He's being very brave and taking a lot of pain."*

I told Samer and Yousef how busy this man was, and how he didn't have the time in his schedule to see a lot of people. I really played it up, telling them how hard it was to get in to see this specialist. Well, we weren't going to see this doctor at all!

Meanwhile, still in Dubai, we were pressured to hurry up and get to Germany for the biopsy. I wondered how I would get my child there – and what he would go through to get cured.

At this point, we didn't know anything except what the doctors had already told us: they suspected Yousef had Ewing's sarcoma, which is a malignant, small, round, blue cell tumor. It is a rare disease of the bone or soft tissue. It most commonly occurs in the pelvis, femur, humerus, ribs or collarbone. Of course, we all Googled Ewing's sarcoma. There is so much information on the net, and that's great, but you tend to find the worst cases and the horror stories. I had to keep in mind that every individual responds differently to treatment; that each case is unique. Anyway, without the biopsy, nothing was for certain. We had no choice but to wait until then, and there was no point in getting upset by what we read on the internet.

For me to stay mentally and physically strong, I decided to keep focused and take each day as it came and make it the best I possibly could. Many people were calling to speak to me, and I was so grateful, even though I couldn't answer all the calls or questions. It was exhausting to repeat everything over and over.

I wrote to Suzie,

"God knows best. Whatever I'm given or not, I'm so grateful for. If I don't manage to speak to you, please just keep Yousef in your prayers. Once I know more, and we've reached where we're going, I'll keep you updated."

In spite of my resolutions, the night before we left for Germany, I stood in my bedroom with my friends around me feeling anxious. I thought we had a doctor and a plan, and I tried to focus on packing. Yet the pressure in my head was incredible.

My husband was unemployed and had been looking for work for some time. We leased our apartment and had to pay the rent a year in advance.

I looked around and felt panic that I might lose my home. I was overwhelmed. I needed my place, my home, my things! At the hospital here in Dubai, at least I knew we could go home at the end of the day. But there would be no "home" once we left the country and went to Germany. All these things were going through my head. Once I left for Germany, I didn't know whether we were ever coming back. There was going to be no income, no certainty. Later, Samer would come back to live in the apartment, but I never would.

I stood in my bedroom that night, surrounded by friends and feeling completely overwhelmed.

"Don't worry," Jill told me, "Your home is going to be here."

"We promise you, your home will be here, and you will come back," they all said.

I wanted to believe them so much. I would miss Dubai, where everything was secure and familiar. I had no idea what we were facing, where we would live, how we would make it – and most of all, how our child would be.

Now I look back, and it seems ridiculous: that I wanted to protect my things – which are just things, after all. It was just because of my confusion and shock – and shows how different I am now.

# CONTAINER VISUALIZATION

Before you continue reading, I invite you to stop for a minute. This visualization is something you can do right NOW to get control over your thoughts and emotions. Therapists use it to help people "contain" overwhelming feelings.

*Don't worry if you're not good at visualization. Do the best you can, and you'll feel the results. Do it over and over, and it will become ingrained. Eventually, you'll be able to instantly and easily have some emotional "breathing room."*

*Go through each step slowly and give yourself time. Maybe you can ask someone you feel safe with read the steps to you. It is great to do this for your child, too.*

Close your eyes and take at least three... deep...slow... breaths.

- Allow all your emotions to rise to the surface.
- Imagine gathering them all up, all your feelings plus all your thoughts.
- See yourself placing all of those emotions in a "container."

*(It can be whatever you like: a gift box, a cardboard box, a tin.)*

- Watch yourself pour all your feelings in and seal the box. Use tape, ribbon, glue, whatever you like. Seal it up tight so that all the emotions are safely locked up in the box. <u>Take your time.</u>
- Now, see yourself put the box on a shelf in a closet.
- Close the closet door and lock it. Step away from the door.
- Look at the door and know the feelings are outside of you, sealed in a box, in that locked closet. You are clear of them for now.
- They are always there if you want to go get them. Maybe you won't.
- Allow the feeling of lightness. Allow yourself to feel relieved. **Breathe.**

## My Notes

# CHAPTER FOUR

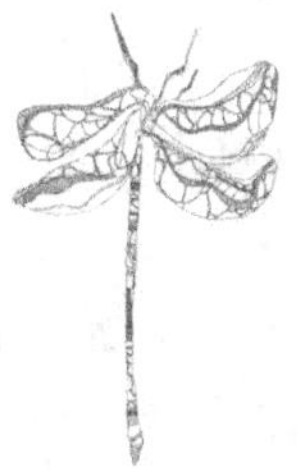

# What Will it Take for Some Happiness to Come?

> *"Difficult roads often lead to beautiful destinations."*
>
> *- Zig Ziglar*

ooking back, I should have taken the advice of the first doctor who told me to "go to your country." We should have flown to Sweden and gone directly to the emergency room and taken it from there. They wouldn't have turned away a young boy. However, I didn't know what consequences that might have had down the road. So, we went another route.

Things were moving very fast. On Friday evening, February 27th, we left the hospital to prepare for our trip to Germany. Salina and Jill had bought Yousef a wheelchair that we could take on the plane. Jill had arranged all the paperwork and made calls about contacts and hotel rooms in Germany. I was amazed at how people are willing to help in a situation like this. A close friend of mine gifted us with business class tickets so it would make it easier for Yousef to travel. His leg was in a cast that stuck straight out, and he would never have fit into a regular airline seat. People also contributed money to help us on our trip.

The two days we had at home before leaving for Germany were mostly happy for Yousef, as people were coming over, and he was just having an ongoing party. Both Samer and I were overwhelmed and still in shock. We were going to travel abroad, taking our child away from his beloved school and home, family, and friends, not knowing what to expect. I had studied German but wasn't fluent. We didn't know what the treatment protocol would be like, what Yousef would be going through or how long we would be gone. The cancer diagnosis alone was overwhelming. We could barely imagine having to leave our home and country too.

On the day we were to leave, which was also my birthday, Yousef woke up at 7:00am in excruciating pain. I gave him some painkillers that took a long while to work. I laid down next to him and sang a lullaby I used to sing when he was a baby. He asked me to tell him the story of the Trouble Tree to help him relax.

At 8:00 am I called Lynn, the school nurse, and asked her if Yousef could pass by before going to the airport to say "goodbye" to his friends. She checked with the principal who agreed.

The doorbell rang, and it was Laith, my son, and Lou, our longtime housekeeper and nanny – who had been with us since my first daughter Salina was 3 years old. We had some Swedish Kanelbullar (cinnamon rolls) together. The smell of freshly baked goods makes me feel happy and homey. I didn't make them from scratch, I bought them frozen from IKEA – I let everyone think I am up at the crack of dawn baking!

We arrived at Safa School at 9.45 am. All the children came down to the front of the school to sign Yousef's cast. Max gave Yousef a lollipop, it was his birthday too - he was turning nine. Rayan told me it was her mum's birthday as well. In the midst of all this upheaval, there were things to celebrate: friends, family, birthdays. We took pictures with everyone, said goodbye and got back into the car and left for the airport.

Yousef was extremely sad, though glad to have all his friends' names on his cast.

He didn't want to speak during the drive, and he asked me to be quiet too. I felt his pain in my heart. I asked myself, what will it take for some happiness to come?

Salina and Jill were driving behind us. Samer, Laith, and Lou were waiting for us at the airport. Only Nathalie wasn't with us as she was in London, at University. She would be the first one to come to Germany, though. I worried that she felt bad about being so far away.

We arrived at the airport, and we checked in easily. Laith pushed Yousef around in the wheelchair until we got to the gate, then it was time to say goodbye to our beautiful family. Until we meet again, I thought. It was so hard to keep the tears from coming. I was flooded with so many feelings about leaving. They were being very brave, but I am very close and connected to my children, and I could feel their sadness as they watched their sick little brother and me leave for another country. No one had any idea what was to come, but they knew I wouldn't be able to be there for them for a while - I couldn't hug them or care for them or make them feel safe. My eldest, Salina told me not to worry, but to take care of Yousef.

"We'll be fine," she said. "Don't worry about us."

I reminded myself that crying would not make anything better – not for me or them. I reminded myself that my thoughts, feelings, and emotions are all in my head. I could not choose the circumstances around us, but I could choose my reaction. I made a choice right then that it would be best for all of us to focus on the NOW. I can still see myself saying goodbye to them, and there are plenty of emotions that come up. I am not unfeeling, but I chose to manage my feelings to help take better care of all of us. Yes, I am their mother, and it is my job to keep the family together and protected, even though they are mostly grown up - it doesn't matter. But, I reminded myself that Lou, our longtime nanny who had become a true member of our family, would be there as always. I knew that Salina had Jill, now her mother- in- law and our friend who had been in our lives since Salina was just a baby. I knew my children had people to support them. I knew this wasn't "goodbye" forever and that my most important mission was to care for my youngest, who was facing the fight of his young life. Now it was time to care for him.

I wanted us all to be together on this flight, so I prayed and wondered what it would take for Samer to be upgraded to business class so that he could sit with Yousef and me. After we parted from our family, we went to the airline's lounge, and I had to ask if my husband could come sit with us. Yousef and I had business class seats which gave us access to the lounge, but Samer didn't.

"OK but only this time," I was told.

It amazes me how some people need to let you know how important they are – all because they have the power to grant you entry to a lounge. Never mind the child in the wheelchair in front of them is heading for cancer treatment and just wants to sit beside his father and mother.

We all got in and found a comfortable place to sit. Yousef was exhausted, and he fell asleep. When he woke up from his short nap, he asked for something to eat, so I got him pasta with tomato sauce and some unhealthy doughnuts and cookies.

After some time, he wanted to use the bathroom, and luckily, it was wheelchair-accessible, unlike many other places. Dubai is not yet entirely accessible, though it is getting more so now.

As the time came to board the plane, I kept asking myself "what would it take for Samer to get upgraded to business class?" It shook me a little when he wasn't. But I tried to stay in the state of asking questions. I wondered, "What else might be possible during this journey?"

We faced a little challenge getting Yousef on board, but we managed, and he settled in and felt secure. This is something he had been thinking about since we told him that we had to fly abroad, but it worked out OK.

We ordered our food. When he ate his soup, I could see he really enjoyed it, and he felt at ease. The flight was smooth, and once we got off the plane, we were met by a nice young guy whom Jill had arranged to help us to get through immigration and customs in Germany. He then drove us to our hotel through the cold and dark night. I still thought we were on our way to Heidelberg. Yousef was very tired by the time we got in the car. We drove for over two hours to Karlsruhe, which is south of Frankfurt. We didn't realize when we stopped at our hotel that the hospital was still another 30 minutes away. Our driver told us that the next morning a *different* man would come and pick us up and take us to the hospital Städtisches Klinikum Karlsruhe fur Kinder. I was looking forward to meeting the doctor in Heidelberg that I had researched and built up so much to my husband and son.

One bright spot was that Jill had managed to book us into a small hotel, Erbprinz, in the town of Ettlingen. When we arrived, we were thrilled to find a quaint, family-run hotel, which would become a comfort and our home away from home for the next three months. I went to sleep confident that once we got to that hospital, we would be in good hands, and hopefully, have some ideas of what was going on with Yousef by the end of the next day.

www.erbprinz.de

Looking back on that trip, I think about how lucky I am to be Yousef's mother. He was so tired and in pain, but he didn't complain. Maybe he didn't even have the words to talk about it. I believe Yousef understood on one level but didn't on another – he was only a child, after all.

## HOW TO MAKE DECISIONS

1.  For the first few days, and maybe even weeks, you are in a state of shock. You might not be taking in the air you need to think clearly and function well. **What might taking a deep breath do for you right now?**

2.  You may feel that what you're hearing is unbelievable. (I couldn't grasp it at first, and I still get emotional just remembering that time, and maybe I always will.) **What would help you understand better?**

3.  There is a lot of pressure to hurry up, make a decision, give an answer, choose a doctor or procedure. Don't decide anything at this very moment. Breathe. You could ask, as I did: **"What would you do if it were your child, doctor?"** And, another good question: **"Thank you. When do you need to hear my decision?"**

4.  If you feel alone or not able to cope, **who do you want to help you?** If that person is not around, there are people who can support you. Even I can support you through the words in this book.

5.  None of your feelings are "wrong." You might have to grieve, get angry, feel alone, frightened, burdened, hopeless, confused, desolate, faithless, faithful. Whatever you

feel, it is normal. Trust me. **What do you feel?**

6. **How might your feelings help you understand your child's feelings?**

7. None of your needs are "wrong." If you need a night's sleep, some more time with the doctor, a change of clothes, help with a fussy baby, it's OK. Getting your needs met helps your sick child. **How (who) can you ask for what you need?**

8. **What else do you need?** If you need to cry and not have someone interrupt you or tell you "there, there, it'll be all right," TELL THEM. You have permission to ask someone to hug you. You have the right to tell someone all you need is reassurance or a listening ear.

9. Yes, there is an urgency to make decisions, and get your child into treatment. Usually, you have a day or so. Talk to someone, ask questions. But no matter how much advice you get from people in your life or on the internet, it'll never be enough, you will never hear the perfect answer, and you will have to choose things on your child's behalf. **How will you know when you know?**

10. You can change your mind, get a second opinion, or ask for other options, or have the

doctors talk more slowly so you can decide with a clear mind and calm heart. **<u>What might be possible with another opinion? What might you learn if you wrote it down, drew a picture or sat down when s/he spoke with you?</u>**

11. Write it down. Take notes on what the doctors tell you. Start right now on the next page. Write down questions. Also, write down personal things: your worst fears, whatever is going through your mind. There is an extra page that you can feel free to rip out after you write on it. Maybe you will rip out the list and take it with you. Maybe you will rip out the page and throw it away because what you have written is too terrible for anyone else to see. Go ahead and do that. It is OK. **What if you became the story-teller? What might you notice that would be helpful?**

12. **What is useful about what you feel?** Feel whatever you feel for as long as you feel it. This is a journey. You can walk it one step at a time. Nothing will seem familiar for a long while. It is OK to feel like a stranger to yourself, to your surroundings. It is normal to feel a little (or a lot) lost.

13. **What would be possible if YOU were well cared for?** Take care of yourself as well as your child. Ask for help in caring for your child, get help for yourself. Even for small things.

# My Notes

# CHAPTER FIVE

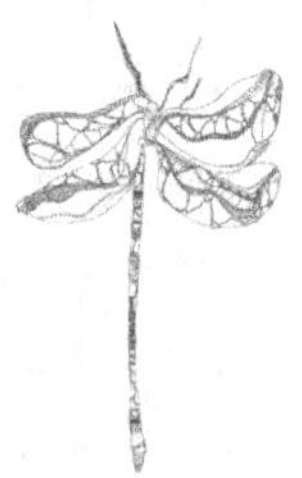

# Now We Know
# What's Next


*"Every day may not be good but there is something good in every day."*

*- Alyce Morse Earl*

The next morning, Monday 2nd March, I woke up hopeful that answers were just a few hours away. In the daylight, I could see the homey touches of the Erbprinz, including the small bouquets of flowers that added color around the hotel.

The hotel has a beautiful spa, and when we were shown around, I imagined sitting in the steam room surrounded by the smell of aromatic oils and relaxing in the sauna and on the lounge chairs on the terrace. It was not to be, and I quickly forgot the hotel even *had* a spa. Samer managed to use it a couple of times, but he was taken aback by a co-ed sauna filled with naked men and women! Samer is a little bit more conservative than the Germans who enjoy their spa days. I used the gym regularly though, keeping up my cardio, strength, and yoga training, though nothing like my old routine at home. In our room, there was a big bathtub where I used to take really hot baths with mineral salts before going to bed. I had to find ways to relax and retreat whenever I could. I remember now how I truly enjoyed those baths and how my body felt a little more relaxed after.

I can't tell you enough how important it is to take care of yourself. Your child is relying on you, and if you can't be at your best because you are over-tired and under-nourished, he or she will suffer. It's easy to become impatient, overwhelmed, and inattentive. Your child needs you at your best, so don't neglect your health or well-being. It is not selfish, it is necessary.

Our room was a suite with kitchenette and a bath with a door wide enough for the wheelchair. Though I couldn't let Yousef take a bath, I'd sponge him from the tub to give him the benefits of the soothing salts.

We weren't used to the cool temperatures of Germany after the sun of Dubai, not that it would matter much in the coming weeks and months as we barely left the hospital or our hotel room. We would explore the town of Ettlingen as time went on – though not with Yousef. His leg would stay in a cast that stuck straight out, making traveling awkward, and as he began his chemo treatments, he felt less and less well.

Ettlingen is a picturesque and historic little town lined with classical style buildings and cobblestone streets. Under other circumstances, it would be a nice place to visit, and I still hope to go back one day.

That first morning, I remember getting up early and having a nice breakfast together. A taxi picked us up at 2:00 pm to take us to the hospital. We reached the hospital 30 minutes later – a longer drive than I expected, but I dismissed any doubts I had.

When we arrived at the Kinder Klinikum, a man named Wael met us. He would become such a help to us. He spoke Arabic and German and would be our interpreter. He took us in to see Dr. Peter Schmittenbecher, who was a professor and head of surgery. Right away, we found out that he doesn't do the sort of operation Yousef would need. That frustrated and confused me. What were we doing here, then? He said they treated kids in their children's oncology ward, but some children had to leave to have surgery elsewhere and returned later to finish their chemo. It seemed like a very confusing process. And I was already confused enough! What would it take to get some answers?

I had been eager to meet the doctor I had heard such good things about, and who I had told Yousef about with such excitement. I was sure he would have answers for me. So, I wanted to talk to <u>him.</u>

"Do you work with Dr. Ho?" I asked.

"Who?" Dr. Schmittenbecher said.

"You don't know Dr. Ho?" I said.

He had no idea who I was talking about. I was shocked and didn't know what to say. I thought, surely this must be an associate of Dr. Ho's. Were we in the wrong place? No, because they had Yousef's name – they'd been waiting for us. He didn't know who Dr. Ho was! It would have been funny had my child's life not been at stake.

Dr. Schmittenbecher got right to business and said he wanted to see Yousef's leg. He'd seen the scans, but he wanted to open up the cast and look for himself. Yousef was worried. His fears were well-founded when the nurse who used a saw to cut off the cast actually slightly cut the skin of his foot in the process! Yousef's fears grew with this accident. Between this and the MRI he'd had a week before, he was getting phobic about tests and treatments. Yousef would go into a state of frantic shock at having to have the cast removed. He is also terrified of needles, which I think comes from a bad experience he had in Dubai. It's not that they did anything wrong, but Yousef never forgot it.

During chemo, I would have to give him an injection in his leg every single day to prevent blood clots because he was getting no exercise. I will never forget the terrible ordeal that first time was. Samer had gone back home for a job interview, and it was just Yousef and me at the hotel. He simply refused to let me give him the shot. It was hours of struggling. I was beside myself, sweating and shaking, anxious and becoming so impatient with my sick little boy. That made me feel like a terrible mother. Later, when his father returned to help with the shots, it got easier. After a while, Yousef got better with shots. We tried to make each shot or procedure into a game that he could win and receive a "prize" for afterward. There are lots of ways to help a child accept the scary parts of treatment. Even simple things to distract the child, like giving him a doll to stab during shots for example. Later, when we were in Sweden, we had a lovely nurse who would get him to sing the 80's song "Staying Alive!" while getting his injections.

When they opened Yousef's cast, I could already see that there was a change in the skin texture of his leg. I was also surprised to see how swollen the leg was. The doctor showed us the MRI, and we could see how the tumor was pushing on the surrounding areas. He told us to come back the next day to check into the hospital – Yousef would go under anesthesia for the biopsy.

Samer and I were really confused and frustrated. It felt like things were up in the air. We had been looking forward to seeing a different doctor in Heidelberg, and now we had Dr. Schmittenbecher, who could only do the biopsy! We'd have to go to *another* hospital for the operation. Had things changed or had I misunderstood from the beginning? I spoke to my daughter Nathalie, and she promised to look into what had happened.

Wael was very sweet and offered us a ride back to our hotel. While driving, both Samer and I thought it would be better if we could have a room somewhere closer to the hospital.

After we got settled back into our hotel room, Samer went out and tried to find something for us to eat, but when he returned, neither Yousef nor I had an appetite. I didn't even feel like talking to anyone. Yousef Skyped with Nathalie, and when he was finished, he just handed me the phone. I ended up talking to her about what happened, and it felt good when she listened. Finally, we went to bed, and Yousef had a rather good night's sleep under the circumstances. Often, during this time, I would tell

Yousef the "Trouble Tree" to help him relax and fall asleep. It can be the most wonderful bedtime story and brought my son so much comfort. I've included it here for you.

## *The Trouble Tree*

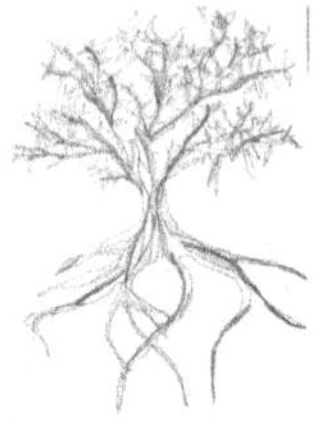

*(This is Yousef's and my version)*
*Read this slowly and quietly to your child, pausing at the end of each sentence. If it is comfortable for your child to take some deep breaths, you might encourage them to do so before you begin.*

*Close your eyes.*

*Imagine you're standing in a big field.*

*The grass is high, and you can see a little path and you follow this path…*

*The sun is shining, and there is a breeze, so you can feel the grass moving.*

*There are beautiful flowers growing in the field: blue, yellow and a few red flowers popping up here and there.*

*As you walk down the path in the field you touch the high grass with your hand... kind of stroking it and it feels so soft -- almost tickling your palm...*

*As you continue walking, you see a forest at the end of the field. So green and thick the forest is.*

*You reach the forest and step in. It is much cooler here. It's almost magical when you step in. And as you look up, the trees are so tall, and it feels much cooler.*

*You can see the blue sky and the trees are moving slowly almost like they're dancing. And you hear the birds singing. Amazing how relaxed and comfortable it makes you feel.*

*As you continue, you're happy skipping along the path. Bending down and seeing beautiful blue berries, and you taste them, and they're delicious.*

*You continue to walk deeper and deeper into the forest. Suddenly, you come to a big wooden gate, it looks very old.*

*You look at me, and I say you can open the gate. You step up on the gate and reach for the metal latch on top and open it.*

*You still stand on the gate, so you ride with it as it opens. I walk past it, and you close it behind us. Then we continue to walk, until suddenly, we see a BIG tree. It looks like it's almost glowing.*

*We walk closer, and you look at me with questioning eyes. I explain that this is a special tree: a Trouble Tree. Here you can leave all of your worries and troubles behind.*

*Now think of all the troubles that you have met with today, and one by one hang them on the branches of the tree.*

*Let me know when you've taken out all the things from your mind that troubles you.*

*(When your child tells you he has hung all his troubles up, continue:)*

*Good. You can now walk away from all of those things that had been bothering you.*

*We walk on another path, and after we have walked a little, we turn around and look at the tree.*

*There is the tree, and all your troubles are hanging there. They seem far away.*

*We continue to walk, and all of a sudden, we reach the same gate, and you open the gate, and I walk through, and you close the gate behind us.*

*We continue to walk on the path, it feels so nice and light as we walk. We can still hear the birds singing and the leaves rustling in the wind. We reach the field where we started, and it's so beautiful with all the flowers.*

*Stay in this safe and peaceful place for as long as you like.*

Yousef is usually asleep after he has hung all his troubles on the tree. There is no right or wrong way to tell this story. Adapt it any way you like. Maybe your child would like to add something to make the story his or her own.

## My Notes

## CHAPTER SIX

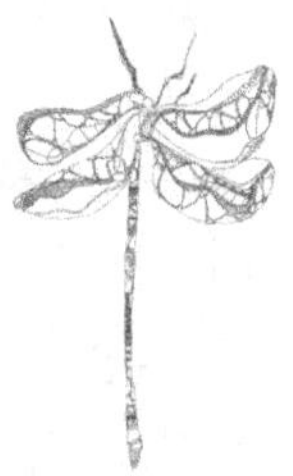

# This Is How It Is

---

*The thoughts we choose to think are the tools we use
to paint the canvas of our lives.*

*– Louise Hay*

---

On Tuesday 3rd March, we woke up and went downstairs and had breakfast. Yousef had a good appetite; he ate an omelet, a sandwich, and drank some hot chocolate. He was a little worried about going to the hospital, but there were no problems at check-in, and Yousef got a light and modern room he seemed comfortable in. The nurses were very accommodating and kind. While Yousef had some tests done, Samer went out with Wael to see the area around the hospital.

I asked a nurse about the activities they had for the kids. She told me about a playroom just next door, and a house outside, staffed by volunteers, where patients' siblings could go and play.

"Maybe I could volunteer there for a few hours if Yousef will be staying long," I wondered aloud.

The nurse just looked at me. I had no idea what Yousef was about to go through. I thought I could volunteer, keep up with my fitness routine, maybe even do some personal training. I didn't realize that cancer was about to completely disrupt life as I knew it. Although, I guess it already had.

I was trying to bring a little normalcy to my life by thinking I could continue some of my regular activities. Later, the same nurse I'd spoken to earlier came back to see me.

"Do you know about the Eltenhaus?" she asked.

I thought she was talking about a home for elderly people, but Elten is "parent" in German.

"Do you think I should volunteer there?" I asked.

"No," she said, "That's where the other parent can stay as only one parent may stay in the hospital room at night."

I looked at her, not understanding. Now I wonder what she must have thought of me – a mother looking to leave her child's side during his worst days to go off and volunteer! But, I imagine most parents walk in like I did, completely unaware of what was about to crash down around them.

Samer went to see the Eltenhaus, and when he came back, he said it was okay. Later, we took the short walk from the Kinder Klinikum together to see it. Parents could have a small private room and a bathroom with a shared kitchen and living room. I saw it as a little miracle: just what we had asked for the day before! How does it get better than this? I thought.

We returned to the hospital, and the oncologist, Dr. Leipold, as well as Dr. Schmittenbecher came in to see us. Dr. Leipold confirmed there was a tumor in Yousef's leg, and he said he'd only know what treatment route to take once the biopsy came back in about 10 days. But he could already tell us this: it would be a long course of chemotherapy. Outpatient, every three to four weeks, for a year. He talked about a similar case he had 3 years ago.

"That boy had his cast removed after 6 weeks," he said.

He said it like this was record time, but Yousef was horrified. Six weeks without walking around? How long without football? As it turned out, Yousef wouldn't be quite as lucky as that other boy.

Dr. Schmittenbecher explained that he'd do the biopsy but not the surgery. It was a delicate operation, and only a specialist could do it. He had a lovely way of explaining it all to Yousef. For the biopsy, he used an analogy of exploring a village to see who is living there.

"Before you know how to treat the residents, you have to meet them, and see what they are like," he said. What he meant was until he knew the type of cancer Yousef had, he wouldn't know the best form of treatment to give him.

Yousef had his biopsy on March 4th, under anesthesia. I cannot describe the feeling of walking away as my child was put to sleep, not knowing if I would see him awake again. It is the most difficult thing for a parent to do, I think. I had to watch him being wheeled away, trusting that others would take care of him for me – that he would go to sleep peacefully and wake up again to look into my eyes.

After the biopsy, Yousef was in terrible pain – he hunched down over his leg as if protecting it. Bone pain is supposed to be the worst type of all. He was given a spinal, and he could click for morphine whenever he needed it.

Dr. Leipold came to see us days later after the biopsy had confirmed the diagnosis. He told us that Yousef didn't have Ewing's, but rather, osteosarcoma of the femur, and he had to start chemo immediately. Now he could be more specific about the treatment. He said that first there would be 6 sessions of chemotherapy, which would take about three months, and then there would be an operation to remove the tumor. Following that, if the leg was clear of cancer, there would be another round of chemo and possibly further surgery or procedures for the leg. He said that amputation was a possibility.

We were all in a state of shock, standing there, practically with our mouths open. We'd had no idea. I tried to ask if there were any other ways to treat it.

"This is how it is," the doctor said.

"Will you do the operation here?" I asked, although Dr. Schmittenbecher had already explained this to me.

"No, we don't perform that surgery here, but you will come back to this hospital and continue chemo for another 12 sessions afterward."

He couldn't tell us how long the process would take because they didn't know how Yousef would react to the medicines. You have to be well, have a good blood count, no fever or infection before they will allow you to start the next round. It can stretch out treatment indefinitely if the child has a reaction, infection, or low platelet count. In the case of a child with osteosarcoma, you have to bombard the cancer with strong intravenous drugs; they want to take no chances of the cancer recurring. It would be a difficult time, and Dr. Leipold did not sugar-coat it. I was thinking, "Hello! Can we talk about this?" but it definitely was not a two-way conversation.

I don't know what I was expecting, but I was so shocked with the medical system. It seemed it wasn't about healing the patient. Chemotherapy was the only thing they were offering. I wondered what will that do to this little boy? How will his body be afterward? And I remembered with a jolt, the doctor had said there was no guarantee his leg could be saved. I had so many questions, but NO doctor could answer them.

Things were moving so fast – I wanted to ask whether there wasn't something else we could do – shouldn't we look for alternatives? I was thinking this is a child we're talking about. What will be the long-term effects of these drugs? How will he manage all of this? Personally, I had always said if it were me, I wouldn't do chemo. I believe cures should come from the ground – and I look for alternatives whenever I can. But this was my child. I wanted to do the best thing for him, but I felt I was signing my son over – to a process I had never had good feelings about. It was terrifying, not like anything I had ever felt before. But there were not a lot of choices, at least as the doctors presented it. They kept saying "quickly, quickly." And because it is my son, I could not take any chances. I believe that when you are faced with something, you have to make up your mind and follow through.

Another aspect of all of this was how long we'd be gone from home. If the doctor's schedule was right, we would be out of the country from February through to the end of November. This was *months* longer than I had ever imagined. As it turned out, we'd never go home again. If someone had told me *that,* I wouldn't have believed it.

After the doctor left, Yousef broke down. He cried and cried and asked so many questions:

"I won't be able to walk for a year?"

"No, that's what the doctor said," I said.

"What about school?" PE? Swimming? FOOTBALL?" he cried.

I felt terrible for him. His whole life had just been taken away. He was so upset, he just crashed and slept. I couldn't do anything to help him or promise anything to make it better for him. That night, I went back to the hotel, and Samer stayed at the hospital. I skyped with Nathalie and didn't go to sleep until 1:00 am.

"I don't want this!" I kept saying.

She promised she would look into alternatives for Yousef, telling me to wait and not to accept the protocol the doctor had described. But it felt as if I didn't have a choice, and I was not going to gamble with my child's life.

Later, I had the chance to speak to the woman who coordinates the Eltenhaus and serves as a support to parents there. I told Claudia about how I wished for alternatives.

"You don't have another choice," she said. "You're in the system, you can't take your son out. It doesn't matter whether you're German or not. Another mother refused to sign the paperwork, but she finally did – you do not NOT sign it."

I finally accepted that chemo would have to happen, but I was also going to do whatever I could that would be natural and not harmful. For example, I used a form of energy healing on Yousef during and after chemo, putting my hands on him and asking that his body would take what it needed and dissipate the rest, releasing the toxins and negative effects of the drugs. I just asked God to please let his body heal and let go anything harmful.

One time a nurse came in during one of my treatments. At first, I didn't know how she would react, but she said,

"Whoa, the energy in this room is amazing!"

Later, I found out that she is a Reiki practitioner. Whatever anyone thought, if it's going to make him feel better, and I am calm when I do it, then it's not making anything worse!

I also firmly believe that prayers and supplications, which anyone can do, have an effect. I do believe God is beyond whatever we can imagine. God knows what I need even before I do. I believe in destiny, but I can still do something to help change the experience for myself and other people around me. I can choose to be positive, to bring light and hope to a situation. To help my child see the positive side, to keep him focused on happy things, things to be grateful for. I believe that good words and good works create good energy around us. I have a strong faith, and I think it helps me accept difficult things. I am also a firm believer in what Louise Hay said, *"I do not fix problems. I fix my thinking. Then problems fix themselves."*

Trying to look at it all in the positive, I kept asking myself questions like, what will it take for Yousef to be totally cured after the whole process? What will it take for his body to heal with ease and joy?

Of course, I still had concerns. There would be so many tests with dyes and contrasts and so many times when Yousef would have to go under anesthesia. It worried me to see him go under that many times. He was so loaded up with chemicals, and no one knows the long-term effects of these substances. Some of them haven't even been around for very long. Like everyone else, we will have to wait and see.

Yousef was so pumped with medicine and felt so sick during treatment, that to this day, there are foods he won't eat.

"Mamma, don't give him his favorite foods when he is so sick, or he'll never eat them again. You'll spoil them for him forever," my daughter Nathalie recommended.

I am glad I took her advice. Yousef still likes sushi – his favorite.

It was Nathalie who felt the most distant from us and removed from everything that was going on with her little brother. She was in London finishing up her studies at University when we found out Yousef had cancer, and she had wanted to fly to Dubai right away. Unfortunately, there just wasn't time. She was the first to come join us in Germany though, and it was wonderful to have her – and it cheered Yousef up so much, even if he couldn't always show it.

Nathalie and I went out shopping one day, trying to think of ways to make Yousef feel better and help him through his upcoming treatment. We bought loads of gifts, small and large. One was a big jar filled with glass marbles of different sizes. We wrapped the gifts and made small cards. We gave them to Yousef every time he had to have medicine, injections, or procedures. It was an incentive, something for him to look forward to. We kept it up after Nathalie went back to London, and I think it helped remind Yousef that she was still supporting him in spirit.

## Centering Yourself

**What would it be like to take a few moments to yourself during difficult days? What if you could intentionally put some distance between you and out-of-control thoughts in your mind? What might be possible?**

Close your eyes and put your hands on your face.

Breathe.

Feel your face in your hands.

Put your hands on your body. Feel your body under your hands.

Breathe.

Feel your feet on the ground. Allow all of the excess energy and worry flow out of your body through your feet into the ground.

Now you are fully here. Aware. Ask yourself:

**What can I do to make it better today than yesterday?**

Breathe.

## Alternatives

Any alternative treatment you try, whether it is diet or herbal or other protocol, can have an effect on doctor-prescribed chemotherapy. There could be an interaction or contraindications with chemo drugs, or the alternative might have side effects of its own.

Is there a way to use alternatives alongside conventional treatments? At first glance, it seems that people either go full-on with conventional treatment or they go entirely alternative, using herbs or supplements, radically changing their diet, starting spiritual practices, and making lifestyle changes. Looking at it more deeply, I found out lots of people combine mild alternatives or lifestyle changes with chemotherapy, surgery, or radiation. The change might simply be drinking more filtered water to flush the chemicals out of their bodies, or they might begin meditating for relaxation.

Be sure your doctor knows about any lifestyle, diet, supplementary, or other changes you make to your child's regimen as he or she goes through treatment. Check with your healthcare providers before giving the child anything that hasn't been prescribed, even vitamins or over-the-counter medications.

I cannot speak about the effectiveness of alternative treatments because we did not go that route. After the phase of active treatments, I started using some alternatives, however.

## Lemon Water

The idea behind lemon water is that it alkalinizes the body, which is often acidic from toxins and poor diet. It's a good source of vitamin C, aids digestions, and helps prevent kidney stones. Drinking it with warm water first thing in the morning can help flush the digestive system and help rehydrate the body. Chemo tends to make the body extremely alkaline, so it isn't recommended to use lemon water during chemotherapy.

## Himalayan Salt

Some believe this is the purest form of rock salt. Its pink color comes from its iron content. You can ingest it or bathe in it, and it is known to contain 84 different minerals that are found in a healthy body, which balance and detoxify. Some people point out that a few of those minerals are radioactive, but not in amounts that can harm you. Himalayan Salt is said to have a high vibrational energy, which is thought to be healing as well.

## Wheat Grass

According to one of the "classic" books about Wheat Grass use, Ann Wigmore writes,

"While wheatgrass juice helps to build immunity, its beneficial effects range much further. Preliminary studies have identified a number of substances in wheatgrass juice that are formidable anti-cancer agents.

One of these is called abscisic acid."

This is a plant hormone, known to "prevent seeds from germinating until environmental conditions are just right." According to Wigmore, research has found that even small amounts of abscisic acid are deadly to any form of cancer.

Another potent contributor to wheatgrass's anti-cancer effects is vitamin B17, laetrile.

Wigmore writes,

"While laetrile as a cancer treatment is still hotly debated (in the US), the facts speak for themselves: the modern…diet contains about 400 times less vitamin B17 than the diet of the natives in countries where the incidence of cancer is very low."

In general, Wigmore recommends wheatgrass as a medicine, tonic, and regular adjunct to your diet for everyone, it's natural benefits include an increased shine of your hair to healing chronic and serious illnesses such as cancer. (See The Wheatgrass Book, Ann Wigmore, Avery Press, 1985.)

## Cannabis Oil

You can find lists of studies showing that cannabis oil cures cancer among other diseases, including diabetes and fibromyalgia. Serious research is ongoing, and preliminary findings are that cannabis oil has several medicinal properties. It can be administered in several ways and is generally well-tolerated by patients. For more information, see www.cureourown cancer.org (among other sites) for more information.

*My Notes*

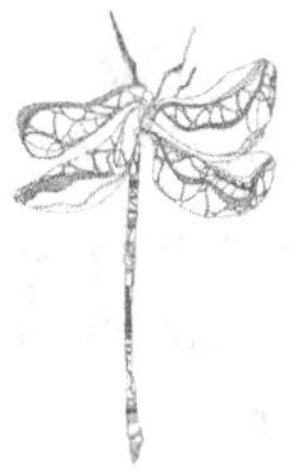

# What Did I Know?

---

*The challenges in our lives are there to strengthen our convictions. They are not there to run us over."*

— *Nick Vujici*

---

Yousef's treatment finally began on March 20th. Looking back now, I realize we didn't know <u>anything.</u> We had no concept of what was going to happen. I didn't think about the future - we were just going along and following directions; following the treatment. All we knew for sure was we could not wait. There was no time to waste.

We expected six treatments, followed by the operation, then 12 more rounds of chemo after that.

We found out the UK, Northern Europe, and the US all follow the same protocol.

We got all of the statistics about osteosarcoma and the outcomes from this protocol compared to others. I found out that it is more common in boys, affecting about 3% of children. It has about a 70% survival rate. I was grateful that Yousef didn't have any metastasis, though I did not know this at the outset. They confirmed it after his operation in July. They had to "decalcify" the bone in order to confirm that it had not spread.

We found out first-hand how many things could delay treatment. For Yousef, it was high white cell counts, fevers, low platelets, and infections. As bad as the chemo was, the idea of operating on his leg was so severe to me that it was hard to grasp. They would be cutting into his *bone!* And we still hadn't chosen the surgeon who would be performing the operation. We didn't know our alternatives, and different people were telling us different things about what hospital would be best to treat a child's osteosarcoma, which is rare.

One thing at a time. Chemotherapy.

On March 20th Yousef went under anesthesia to have his port put in. They put it into his rib area, not his shoulder as we found was more common in other countries. When they found the port at his rib when we came to Sweden, they were surprised to see it there.

The same day as the port placement, we moved to the oncology floor where Yousef began his treatment. There was no break for him, and the first round of chemo was the worst because they start with a very high dose of Methotrexate for 24 hours, followed by a "flush" of his system with Leucovorin, a compound similar to folic acid. It isn't a chemotherapy drug in itself, but it's been used for many years in combination with chemo drugs to enhance the anti-cancer effects of some drugs and reduce the side effects of others.

Yousef was OK the first day, but on the next, he began vomiting and having diarrhea. It was awful – I had never seen anything like it. At the same time, he had to take antibiotics, which he couldn't swallow – he didn't want to swallow anything for fear of vomiting and because he felt so nauseated.

We would later find out that not every country handles antibiotics this way, expecting the child to take them orally even when they can't keep anything down. In Sweden, they only gave Yousef antibiotics when he had a fever, to beat an infection.

It was a nightmare to watch how sick he was, but the nurses were excellent – capable and compassionate. As it was all new to me and I was in shock, the night nurse stayed in the room next to us.

She was strong and calm. She tried homeopathic pills for the nausea, but once Yousef had started to vomit, nothing could really stop it.

"Is this normal, to vomit so much and to have diarrhea at the same time?" I asked.

"Every child is different," the nurse said.

I know now that Yousef reacted hard to the medicines. I could not believe what chemo did to my son. I was completely unprepared for it. He got three different drugs during the treatment; two in a combination, and one on its own. One would make him more nauseated during the treatment, and another one was easier, with worse side effects after.

Yousef also had a really hard time with thrush or sores that would form on his lips and in his mouth as the chemo took away the natural flora. He had to rinse his mouth all the time; his lips bled, and the pain in his mouth made eating even harder. Once he experienced the sores, he rinsed like crazy to try to prevent them from coming back again. One thing we found that worked well was coconut oil, which he used on his lips and in his mouth. He was so happy with the result that he was really glad to use it.

After that first, hard treatment, the hospital switched to tablets to "flush" the system of chemo drugs. I couldn't believe it when they said they expected us to do this on our own, at "home," which for us was a hotel 30 minutes away! In Sweden, they do the flush in the hospital and won't send you home until the chemicals in the body have been reduced to a certain level. But while we were in Germany, Yousef would be released from the hospital, and we'd go back to our hotel where I would try to give him this medicine every six hours. I would have to wake him and beg and plead with him to take the Leucovorin. I thought I would go crazy. I can still hear how I was told so firmly, in German,

"It is vitally important to give it to him exactly every 6 hours!"

Even Yousef remembers how it was in Germany, "They were very strict there," he says.

I was alone with Yousef since Samer had returned to Dubai for a job interview. There was no one for me to lean on, and Yousef gave me such a hard time. I felt like a terrible mother, because of what I was asking him to do, but also because of how frustrated I would get with him. I wanted to do the right thing and save my son, but I felt I was adding to his suffering. Of course, he was afraid to be sick, and he felt so nauseated that the thought of swallowing tablets was unimaginable. So I was there inflicting daily antibiotics and injections, plus this "flush" every six hours. It was exhausting. I was finding out for myself just how tough the treatment protocol for osteosarcoma is. To handle side effects,

Yousef was sent "home" with homeopathic pills for nausea and herbal tea for both rinsing his mouth and drinking to prevent nausea. I remember it was sage and chamomile and *not* very effective.

It was ironic to me that in the two years prior to this, Samer had only worked on and off, and then when his child gets sick, he gets called for a job interview in Dubai. Samer hesitated about leaving us, but I encouraged him to go. I knew that he thought it was his role to support us financially. It was hard without him, but we sometimes clashed because of how we approached things, so looking back, it was for the best that he left. Besides, the pressure of the enormous expense of treatment weighed on him, and I knew he had to do something to feel useful. I think Yousef is still a little angry that his father was not there. We still don't live together since Samer can't work in Sweden where Yousef and I live now.

Samer came back to Germany after the first treatment was over. Yousef woke up on the third day and said I'm feeling "good," as if he had woken up from a horrible three-day nightmare. Samer took over doing the shots in Yousef's leg, and it was better for all of us. He left again in April, and after that, it was just Yousef and me again, so I couldn't walk away, even for a short time.

One day, a few weeks after treatment had begun, Yousef came back from the hospital with his father after bloodwork. His blood had to be tested regularly to be sure he was healthy enough to continue treatment.

"Mamma," he said, and hugged me. He held me hard and was quiet. "My hair is coming out when I put my hands through it."

"That's okay your hair will grow back, my darling," I said. I knew this was very hard for him, but I didn't want to make it a big deal. He went to play his new Wii U game. Yousef tells me I'm saying that wrong, that it's just the Wii, but whatever. And, he reminds me that it wasn't Laith who gave it to him. It was a father of another patient, a little girl, who just came up to Yousef out of the blue and gave him the game. It reminds me how cloudy some of my memories are, and it touches me that a stranger would give my son this expensive toy because he thought it might make him feel happier.

That afternoon, I made mujaddara for Yousef and Samer with cucumber and yogurt salad. Mujaddara is rice, lentils, and onions cooked together to a soft consistency, like risotto. This was easy for Yousef to eat. While I made the food, and Yousef was in the other room, Samer and I talked.

"I don't know what to say to him about his hair," Samer said.

"I don't want him to see us get upset about it," I said. "Then he'll just get *more* upset."

That afternoon, we were waiting for Salina, who was arriving from Dubai. She had landed safely, but they had lost her luggage, and she was still at the airport, hoping it was on the next flight. I went to meet her at the train station– her luggage still hadn't turned up. What a crazy inconvenience in light of everything else we were going through! It was so great to see my beautiful daughter. When we got to the hotel, Yousef was happy to see her, too.

The next day, Yousef didn't want to come downstairs to eat breakfast with us. I supposed it was because of his hair, but maybe he didn't feel well enough to come. Later, we all went to the hospital for his blood test, and on our way he pulled at his hair, watching it come out in horror. While we waited at the hospital, he pulled loads of hair out, pulling faster and faster, so in shock. Salina spoke to him quietly, telling him we could shave his head later. Samer had expected this day to come. He'd shaved his head already, before returning to Germany, to be in solidarity with Yousef.

In spite of how panicked he seemed, Yousef felt it wasn't such a huge thing YET: Vin Diesel, who he loved, was bald, and anyway, he still had his eyebrows and eyelashes. After you lose those, you look very different, and he was quite self-conscious about that happening.

The rest of the day, Salina and I did ordinary things together: laundry, some shopping, and walking around the town. When we got back, her bags had arrived. We took Yousef to the bathroom and shaved his head. I guess the reality of it was quite a shock, because the next morning, Yousef didn't want to come downstairs to eat breakfast with us because now he was even more self-conscious.

From time to time, we tried to enjoy the sun a little bit. We went down to the lake in Ettlingen, not knowing – having never been told – that chemo makes the skin very sensitive. We should have been more careful. I miss the sun on my face," Yousef said.

The treatments were sometimes really heavy, and as Yousef's body got weaker, the routine was interrupted more and more. Yousef might have a high white cell count, low platelets, fevers, or mouth ulcers. Any of these things would take him off schedule. He was supposed to have one treatment, then another, followed by two weeks' rest.

When the treatments were first interrupted because he wasn't well, I felt anxious to get back on track. But, after a while, I saw it gave Yousef a break, which I decided wasn't such a terrible thing. I dreaded what the chemo did to him when he was in the midst of it.

In Germany, they are very conservative about food, so Yousef's diet was severely restricted. He could take no stone fruit and no raw vegetables; only apples, bananas, pears; only things that were boiled or steamed. He would eat none of the food in the hospital – none! So it was good I could make food in the Eltenhaus. Yousef likes tasty food, but we were told he could only have bland food, which we didn't understand. I had no idea what to feed him. Later, when we were in Sweden, they had a very different philosophy: it is better for the child to eat whatever he wants, as long as he eats. One piece of advice Yousef has: "Let the child eat what they feel like eating!"

We were fortunate that Yousef didn't have to have a feeding tube as some children do. He did lose a lot of weight but avoided the tube.

My children's aunt is very knowledgeable about the macrobiotic approach to diet. She recommended I try it with Yousef, and she gave me a book called <u>The Cancer Prevention Diet</u>. It has loads of information and a guide to different types of cancer. I followed the one for bone cancer.

The Macrobiotic diet is mostly brown rice, boiled like porridge, and was very easy for Yousef to eat. They recommend beginning with just a few basic preparations, such as brown rice, miso soup, a few vegetable dishes, one sea vegetable, and bancha tea. Fish and meat were to be avoided. However, a small amount of white-meat fish may be eaten once every ten days to two weeks if the patient is craving it. Then, day by day, week by week, you can gradually widen the selection of natural foods and introduce new cooking styles. The important thing is to make changes in the right direction. They describe it as building endurance – it's a marathon, not a sprint. Fortunately, there are lots of organic stores in Germany – so we stocked up.

We made adjustments to the macrobiotic diet. For example, yogurt felt cool in his mouth, so though it was not macrobiotic, I gave it to him. Later, I could add beans or lentils to his regular diet, and he likes those things, so it became easier to feed him. I was stricter with him in Germany, following their protocol, but I was concerned when they didn't recommend raw vegetables or fruit. I appreciated the idea in Sweden where they said the child could eat whatever he wanted. But at first, Yousef, remembering the warnings about avoiding certain foods, would protest when we'd offer him something "forbidden." I had to convince him it was OK; that it was better that he eat something.

Chemo had turned him off to so many foods, things that he still won't touch. It was only one lasting reminder of the time he had in between those "I feel good!" days.

# Terrible Thoughts are Normal

*Sometimes we have terrible thoughts. They are part of being human. They are especially likely when things are hard, and we are under stress. It might be that our thoughts surprise or embarrass us. We might think we are "bad" for having them. Or, we might feel ashamed for even thinking them. But, we aren't bad people. We are very normal! Few of us like to admit terrible thoughts, even to ourselves, but I would like to give you permission, if I can, to go ahead and accept what you are thinking. Think the thought, and then let it go. Breathe and see what thought might come next.*

*This is a list of some things we might think…but you might have other thoughts.*

I **hate** this doctor (Or, This doctor is an _________.)

I don't want to do this anymore.

I want to run away.

I just want my old life back.

Maybe my child will die.

Maybe if it is going to be <u>this</u> bad, it would be better if my child died.

I can't stand my husband/wife, I wish they would go away and let me handle this my way.

I wish I could go away and let my husband/wife handle this for me.

What is the reason God has done this to me?

What do these doctors know?

Where is my useless family in all this? Why aren't they helping me more?

I hate my family.

I am never going to speak to __________ again once this is over.

This is never going to end.

I can't take any more.

I can't be there watching when my child __________.

No one cares.

I feel like I'm neglecting my other kids.

My kids will have to just fend for themselves for a while.

I am a bad mother/father.

I caused this illness.

My child/husband/mother/other caused this illness.

If only we didn't __________, then none of this would have happened.

You can also acknowledge and then feel free to let go of any thoughts of:

Anger.

Shame.

Fear.

Guilt.

Grief.

Doubt.

Fill in your own here:

What else? Does your child have terrible thoughts, too? Tell him or her that it's OK and listen if he or she is willing to tell you.

## My Notes

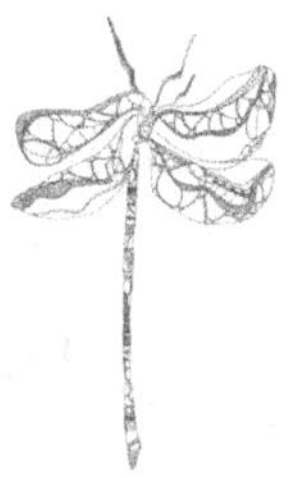

# CHAPTER EIGHT

# Could It Come Back?

---

*"Courage: the most important of all virtues because
without courage, you can't practice any other virtue
consistently."*

*- Maya Angelou*

---

On top of everything going on with treatment, I
was thinking about the surgery Yousef would
need to remove the tumor. I was researching and
searching the internet, getting advice from everyone
I knew as well as calling doctors all over Europe. Dr.
Leipold told us which centers in Europe were skilled
in cancers like Yousef's, so I narrowed down the
hospitals to three: one in the UK, where two of my
kids were, one in Sweden, where I would be in my

homeland (a big plus), and the hospital in Heidelberg – the place I thought was the answer to all my prayers a few months earlier.

I tried every possibility to go to the UK, but when we found out that they wouldn't take us unless we could pay for the surgery ourselves, it was out of the question. I went down the list to Heidelberg to meet with the surgeon there. We traveled between chemo treatments when Yousef felt well enough to go. It is a very beautiful city by the lake; south of Frankfurt. It was spring, and the cherry trees were blooming. It was warmer there than Karlsruhe.

I focused on being positive, making a point of noticing the sights around me. I refused to shut down and be swallowed up by cancer. I imagined we were living in beautiful Heidelberg as Yousef recovered from surgery there.

"OK, I will be alone here, I will live in the hospital, and we will go back to Karlsruhe after the operation," I thought.

The surgeon we met drew a diagram of Yousef's leg and described how she would drill into his femur. Once she saw the condition of his bone, she would decide between an internal or an external prosthetic, which would lengthen the leg bone as Yousef's body grew. She showed us how the mechanism would work.

"I don't want to put that in!" Yousef said.

The doctor explained, until she opened up the leg, she wouldn't know for sure *if* she would be able to put in a prosthetic. Yousef could still be facing losing his leg.

"Oh my God," I said. "We had no idea!"

I was also thinking, "the kid is right here while you talk about cutting off his leg!"

Maybe we should have said something to the doctors about speaking in front of Yousef, but later he told me that he was glad that he was there to hear everything. I am not sure what I would advise another parent about that. It depends on their child's age and maturity. It's also probably something that has to be decided over and over during the process. Some things the child can hear, other things, maybe not.

"Could it come back?" Yousef asked. He was thinking about everything that he had gone through already, and now, a whole new challenge. It was natural for him to wonder: if I go through all this, will you guarantee cancer won't come back?

"Yes," she answered. "It could come back, yes. But, if you think about it, anybody can get sick at any time."

I appreciated her honesty, and personally, I agreed: we can't deny illness or death. But, I don't want to live in that fear, and I didn't want Yousef to either.

With our heads spinning with all the information, we returned to Karlsruhe for another round of chemo. The next two weeks were up and down: Yousef was exhausted, but there were days he could smile. During this round, they gave Yousef Emend before his treatment to prevent the extreme nausea he experienced before. It helped somewhat. Still, he had nausea and terrible mouth ulcers, so he preferred not to eat at all. He also avoided eating because going to the bathroom was also such a struggle with his leg straight out in a cast. In his mind, it was simply better not to eat. I let him have some things that were not strictly on the diet the German doctors had prescribed because I could tempt him with them – to get something into him. I wanted to avoid a feeding tube if we could.

After that treatment, we left the hospital for a break of two weeks, and Yousef's dad returned to Dubai. We didn't see Samer again until August, a long while after Yousef's surgery. It was hard for Yousef to be away from his father, and he didn't understand why he wasn't there for his operation.

I still had to choose the hospital where the tumor would be removed. I contacted friends, acquaintances – anyone, anywhere in the world who might give me some direction. Finally, a friend in

Dubai had her husband (who is a heart surgeon) put me in touch with Dr. Cyril Toma, an oncology surgeon from Austria who works in Abu Dhabi. I can't say enough what help and support Dr. Toma was to me. He recommended we go to Sweden. He said probably the doctors in Heidelberg and in London were very skilled but as important as the delicate surgery, was the follow-up care. Not only would the treatment after the operation take a long time, but then Yousef would need to be followed for more than 10 years afterward!

Ten years. That convinced me to go to Sweden rather than be alone in Heidelberg, in yet another new city, alone, for all that time. I wanted to have the surgery and any long-term care in the same place. I wanted us to settle into some sort of routine in a someplace familiar. If Yousef developed complications or problems in the future, we'd know the language and would have some support. Once I made up my mind, that was it. I was going to Sweden, and no one was going to stop me. The problem was, no one was calling me back.

Dr. Toma spoke to an old professor, a colleague of his in Sweden, who recommended a surgeon: Doctor Otte Brosjö. I had a hard time getting hold of him, and time was crucial. I didn't understand why he wasn't returning my calls. Maybe he was just too busy to do the surgery. The prosthetic device had to be custom-made. Maybe he didn't think it would it be ready in time for Yousef? At this point, I was so determined I was ready to just get on a plane and sit in the ER waiting room.

Feeling desperate one night I called Dr. Toma basically pleading with him. He asked me for Dr. Otte's phone number. The following day Dr. Otte sent me an email. I never asked what Dr. Toma said to Dr. Otte, but whatever it was, I am very grateful!

Dr. Otte is an amazing man. He has a passion for what he does, he works out of conviction. When we met with him, he sat down with us, and he spoke with a casual and positive attitude. He told us everything was going to be fine. He made me feel so calm. He is the kind of doctor who doesn't ask his assistants to do things for him – he does them himself. He still teaches and is part of the Sarcoma Group of Scandinavia.

One of the wonderful things about our decision to have Yousef's surgery and follow-up treatment in Sweden is that here, physiotherapists work with surgeons, making sure that they know exactly how to do rehabilitation and training with the patient post-op. The prosthetic that would be inserted is made to work with a particular machine that slowly lengthens the leg over time. Because these two things operate together, you have to use the same manufacturer for the insert and the machine. Along with the lengthening, Yousef would have physiotherapy to help him learn to balance and walk and regain the strength in his body.

The therapists understand exactly where and how the prosthetic is placed in his leg. Yousef's is very close to his knee, so it is a special challenge to train him. Dr. Otte worked closely with the therapists to find the best way. It truly was a team effort.

I want to note that Dr. Otte, unlike the surgeon in Germany, never mentioned anything about Yousef possibly losing his leg. He ordered the prosthetic, and that was that. Once we decided on the doctor and the hospital, we had to figure out how to get to Sweden and how to pay for everything.

When you have a child who has a life-threatening illness, you worry about him taking his meds, staying on his treatment schedule, and getting him to eat. You are concerned with how he is coping emotionally, and how to take care of yourself and the rest of your family. The last thing you need to think about is how you're going to pay for the treatment and surgery your child needs to get well. I had decided not to worry about the money, but to trust it would come. We were willing to go into debt if necessary and worry about paying it back later. But, hanging over us was the not only the costs but the urgent timing of Yousef's situation as well as Samer's absence and extended unemployment.

If we were living in Sweden, we wouldn't have to worry about paying for medical care, but our situation as ex-pats and non-residents of Sweden meant it was a big concern. The estimate for the surgery was 100,000 Euros or more. That would include ten days in the hospital, but it didn't include any additional expenses if Yousef had to stay longer or if he needed additional hospitalizations because of infections or complications.

To get into the Kinder Klinikum in Karlsruhe, Jill had arranged support for us through a friend who works for a very prominent man in Abu Dhabi. One of my close friends bought us the plane tickets to fly to Germany, and others paid for our stay at the hotel in Ettlingen. All the hospital bills in Germany were settled from abroad.

In order for us to even enter Sweden, a fee was required up front. It upset me that though I'm a Swede and my child is a Swede, I felt unwelcome, and I had to pay an enormous price. People advised me to just go to Sweden and sit in the emergency room, reasoning they wouldn't turn away a child, and the EU has an agreement for emergency care. But I didn't know what the consequences of that might be, and I didn't want to take any chances with Yousef's healthcare.

Fortunately, Samer's uncle paid the hospital fee for us, and since Yousef and I were both Swedish citizens, I knew that once we signed into the country, he'd have same medical rights as any other citizen. The Swedish system is wonderful if you live there. Both parents get paid family leave if there is a sick child, or for the birth of a child. But since I hadn't lived in Sweden for 25 years, I wasn't eligible for any of these benefits.

I wouldn't get sick leave to care for him or non-employment benefits. But, we were able to get some help, and something is better than nothing. I am grateful for that!

At the time, I had no idea how the finances would work out. I didn't know that funds would come from all sorts of people and places. An amazing amount of money was raised from garage sales and fund-raisers, sponsored by Yousef's school and by our friends. Support came pouring in, and I am so grateful, and I intend to pay it forward, in part through this book. When so much is stressing a family, support and generosity are so touching and encouraging, it lifted me up when I was down and gave me hope that all would work out as it should.

A friend of mine had warned me about the bureaucracy in Sweden, but it wasn't as bad as I'd expected. They sent me the papers and I handled everything via mail and phone calls. My friend

Cecilia made calls in Sweden and went to Stockholm's Care for me. She became my guarantor in Sweden.

We'd made up our minds that Sweden was the best place for the rest of Yousef's treatment, we got permission to go, and we had the funding. Now, we had to figure out how to get there. For whatever reason, I had it in my head that we couldn't fly. It would have been less than two hours, but I didn't know how Yousef would cope on the plane, so we decided to drive. It was an adventure I'll never forget – we were on a mission! When someone suggested it was "Mission Impossible," I said no, not impossible. I choose to think like Audrey Hepburn, who said, "I'm possible!"

## Grounding Exercise

If it all feels like it's been too much and your head is spinning, here is an exercise that might help you. Of course you are overwhelmed with information, emotion, personalities, demands, and most of all, anxiety and fear.

So often, we can't integrate everything that is going on around us because we are caught up in our thoughts and feelings. It's OK. If you can ground yourself, and allow that energy to be rooted back to the earth, you will feel better, and clearer.

You may read this to yourself or ask someone to read it to you. Once you know how to do it, you won't need to read it anymore. It will become another tool in your tool belt – available whenever you need it.

If you see your child is struggling, this would be a good meditation to read to him or her.

* * *

First: If possible, sit upright in a chair, with your feet on the ground. Then (once you are seated and comfortable) you can begin.

*Notice how you are breathing. We often breathe only from the very top of our lungs when we are in distress.*

*Just notice for a moment.*

*Feel the shallowness of your breathing.*

*When you are ready, just silently tell your breath, "Slow down. Shhhhh."*

*Allow it to slow. Allow it to deepen. Don't force or even "intend." Just allow.*

*Let your breath sink down and let it take up more space in your diaphragm.*

*Breathe there in that deeper place for a moment or two.*

*Allow your breath to sink deeper into your belly.*

*Now, bring your awareness to your feet on the floor. Feel the contact your soles make with the sock... with the shoe... and finally, with the ground.*

*Imagine that you are breathing all the way from your nose to your lungs, diaphragm, belly, seat, legs, and feet.*

*All of you breathes.*

*All of you is receiving the energy of oxygen and the peace of your breath.*

*Now, imagine that your feet on the floor are beginning to grow roots.*

*The roots drill down past the floor.*

*The roots strongly dig into the earth.*

*They go, deep into the ground, to the very core at the center of the earth.*

*You have roots to this earth now, to this ground that you are connected to.*

*Feel the roots go deep and strong.*

*Allow yourself to feel grounded.*

*All the swirling thoughts and feelings now have roots, too.*

*Feel them all drain right out through your feet. All the negative feelings, the anxiety, questions.*

*Let them go out of your body, into your feet, into the earth, deep into the ground.*

*The Earth holds you, roots you, grounds you. It takes all this and gives you support.*

*As the energy flows from your head and throat and chest and belly, it flows down through your feet and into the earth.*

*Again, feel your feet solid on the floor. Feel the roots going down, anchoring you.*

*You are solid now.*

*You are strong.*

*The energy in you is steady.*

*You are calm.*

*And always, at any time, you may ground yourself like this, and feel the strength that is at the root of your being.*

# A CONVERSATION
# WITH MARCUS' MUM

This interview is with Maria, the mother of Marcus, who was diagnosed with clear cell sarcoma of the kidney in June of 2015. I have translated this conversation from Swedish.

**Me: How has your child's experience with cancer changed you?**

**Maria:** I have always been an Easy-minded person, and it has also colored me in my role as a mother. But when the diagnosis came, and everything fell down on us, I felt my soul was overwhelmed with a severity of the situation . A realization, an insight that my child can no longer have a trouble-free and normal childhood (according to society's general perception). That the everyday life now would be twisted and curbed by hospitals with all of their related unpleasantness that comes with the treatments, the ailments, such as nausea, pain, change in appearance, etc. As a parent, the feeling of powerlessness is the worst. I was supposed to be a caretaker and protector, but I could not help my child to get relief. I couldn't kiss the pain away and make it better. I couldn't wipe away the evil so that my child could continue to play.

This event has made me realize that there is no point arguing or nagging about the small things in life, like loading the dishwasher, or hanging up his backpack when he gets home from school. It is about focusing on the important things in life: to teach my child the importance of how to treat people, the magnitude to love unconditionally, and the understanding that shared joy is double joy. Yes, it may sound corny and cliché, but it's really true. I came to terms that I no longer want to waste my precious energy on nagging and bickering, things that won't improve my relationship with others, or the quality of my life.

At the beginning, I had neither the strength nor the energy to take into account the feelings of anyone other than myself and my son. Then, I could go and squabble with people for the slightest, smallest of things because my patience was non-existent and my jealousy was enormous. The jealousy of other parents who did not have to go through what we were going through. They were able to continue their lives completely untouched. Life was downright so unfair. But I also realized very quickly that there was so much support and love around us from all directions, expected and unexpected. So many showed their support and empathy for what we were going through, and that made us strong and helped us get through it easier than what we thought we would.

**How has your child's experience with cancer changed your perspective on life?**

Where should I start? Life is short and fragile. Everything you've ever taken for granted could be destroyed and become non-existent during the course of one-hundredth of a second. So, as of 9 June 2015 (the day Marcus was diagnosed), I would no longer take anything in life for granted. Every moment, every second is to be enjoyed as if it could not have been better!

Show love to every person in your life, without restraint, and see how much positivity life can bring. To realize that the negativity will never be as big as having to watch your children suffer and not being able to do anything about it. The biggest difference in my life is where I choose to focus my energy on.

I have realized how small and insignificant in the world, but also how loved and important I am to those close to me.

**How has your parenting changed?**

I know that during the early stage, I was somewhat more relaxed (about my expectations and "rules,") and tiptoed around a lot of things, just because there was enough misery as it was. My child should not have to be nagged on further and hear crap from me as a parent now that he already had so much going on and suffering to endure.

But I recovered quite soon from that thought. My child will get through this and become an adult, so I had to do my part and raise him well. He will still grow up to be a good individual with good morals and good values. So, pretty soon, I realized that there was no point in tiptoeing, and the silk gloves came off. Of course, I did my best to try to provide him with the food that he craved, and the entertainment that made life easier as well.

But I never stopped making demands and encourage him to aspire to the best that he could be in the essentials, such as school, health, and attitude toward others.

So really, if you're looking deeper, then my parenting has not changed much, but on the other hand, I have learned to appreciate the moments when everything goes as I hope and want to.

To face a serious, life-threatening situation, whether it is yourself, or someone near and dear to you who's the victim, is never easy, no matter how many times you experience it or how prepared you may think you are. The key is to never lose yourself and let it overwhelm you to such an extent that you lose sight of the difference between good and evil. Being able to receive love and support during the heavy periods, and find the joy in those moments that can provide you with the energy to process the hardship life can bring.

Find your focus and put it on the essentials, as your child's road to recovery, the love you have for each other in the family and amongst friends. The security you can find around you can be your companion when you feel hopeless and when all is overwhelming, and it feels like you will drown in your sorrow. That's when you use the love that's all around you to keep you afloat.

I cannot escape the fact that this will forever change both me as a person but also my child, but we choose to see it as a life lesson, an experience that shows us how we should spend the time we have on earth.

## My Notes

# CHAPTER NINE

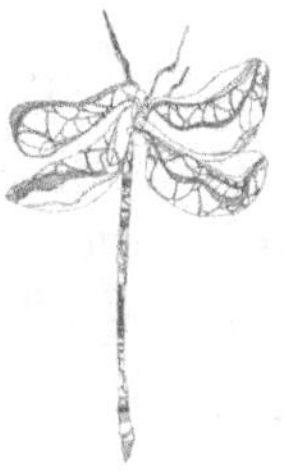

# Escaping To Home



*"Trotzdem Ja Zum Leben sagan means "Yes to life despite everything."*

*– Jurriaan Kamp*

As we got closer to the time of our departure, it got more and more stressful. We were scheduled to start another round of chemo in Sweden on the 1st of June. That's when we were expected on ward Q84, the oncology floor at Astrid Lindgren Children's Hospital in Stockholm. Yousef <u>had</u> to be strong enough to make the long trip. The staff at the hospital in Germany did everything they could to make sure of that. Yousef had had so many setbacks that we weren't sure he would be well enough to even leave the hospital, never mind drive 24 hours through half of Europe! And, on top of everything else, Yousef's passport was due to expire on the 26th of May! I felt like we were illegal immigrants trying to deceive the authorities without the right paperwork, scrambling across borders with a strange man we had paid to smuggle us in! (More about that in a minute!)

There was action and suspense: would we make it in time, or would Yousef's passport expire? We wanted to be in Sweden on the 28th of May to get at least a little settled before we had to report on Q84 -- we were cutting it very close! Losing time would set Yousef back, and we just couldn't afford that.

Before we could even leave, we had so many details to keep track of. I had to make sure all the paperwork was in order for the hospital and the country. I was so relieved that by the time we arrived, Yousef's case had been studied and was really well known by all the doctors there – such a weight lifted! All the oncologists and surgeons on his case were specialists in their fields. I felt it was worth every hardship to be accepted at Astrid Lindgren Children's Hospital. I felt like we'd been hanging between life and death, and then we were told, "you are welcome to come." I kept thinking, now my child is welcome to come to my home country! It felt different from getting the OK to come to Germany.

This was my old home, the place where I was born, and where my child was a citizen. It felt like it was right: a homecoming.

All this time, the doctors and nurses at the Kinder Klinikum were trying to get Yousef strong enough to travel. On May 22nd, he was still in the hospital, and on the 25th, he had to get platelets. He'd reacted badly to getting blood in the past, so they used medication to help his body accept the platelets, to prevent him from getting sick, which would force us to postpone the trip. Everyone knew it would not be easy. It would be 24 hours of straight driving to get to the new hospital. We would drive up through Belgium, Holland, Denmark, into Sweden, then all the way up to Stockholm. I am sure some of the staff at the hospital thought we were crazy to try it.

My husband had said his uncles were coming to drive us on the long trip. That morning, I waited for them to arrive. Finally, I called my husband.

"Samer, where are your uncles?" I asked.

"They are not coming," he said.

"What?!" I couldn't believe what I was hearing.

"Don't' worry," he said, "I found someone else."

"Someone else? Who?!" I asked.

Samer had met a man in Germany and contacted him without me knowing. His mother sent money to pay for this guy and his camper van to drive us all the way to Sweden. Samer thought the camper would be the most comfortable for Yousef in his cast, and Yousef had always wanted to go in a camper, so Samer thought it was a good idea. But we didn't know the driver, and I didn't love the idea of spending 24 hours cooped up in a van with a sick child and a man I'd never met.

"With a total stranger?!" I said.

"Don't worry!" Samer said.

The driver arrived, and we loaded the camper and set out. Yousef was very excited to go, and we both had the feeling that we were on a mission. Yousef slept, but I stayed up. I couldn't stop my thoughts. I barely spoke to the driver; I just wanted to get to Stockholm.

I felt like I was harboring a fugitive since Yousef's papers were about to expire and we were being driven by a man who'd been paid to smuggle us across borders! Would we be pulled over? Would Yousef get sick along the way, and we'd have to stop? That would mean we'd be traveling with an expired passport for sure. In case he got sick, I'd mapped out every hospital along the way so we'd know where to pull off the highway.

I didn't know what would happen. I felt like I was running away and escaping into my own country!

The driver was dedicated to the mission. The poor man only stopped when he absolutely had to –

driving almost continually for 24 hours. I remember he napped once for a short time on the ferry to Denmark and then he asked one other time if I would mind that he rested for 30 or 40 minutes. He was a professional driver, but his stamina was truly amazing!

Most of our friends and family stayed up keeping vigil with us all that night. We texted back and forth the whole time, nobody sleeping, everyone anxious to hear we'd crossed over and were safely in Sweden.

The camper was uncomfortable since Yousef couldn't stretch out to sleep. We'd have been better off in a station wagon!

I will never forget the morning of the 27th driving over the bridge from Copenhagen to Malmö. The sun was coming up over a brilliant blue day, so beautiful, fields full of yellow – grapeseed, maybe? It felt like freedom. We didn't need to worry about the passport, or getting stopped. We were free. Nobody could throw us out now. We were so glad to reach Stockholm and finally arrive at my father and step-mother's home.

It would have been nice to have a different sort of welcome when we got there, but my dad and his wife Runa were nervous about us coming. Yousef felt it too. It wasn't our home, it was my dad's. I really missed my mother so much during this time.

A mother is always a mother. Even if all she had was a shoebox, my children and I would've been welcome. Not that someone does it right or wrong, I just would have done it differently. I would have said to my child, "I am here for you. Stay as long as you want, this is your home." Maybe I am used to Arabic and Mediterranean culture where families are tight; there is so much connection. But my dad and his wife were afraid of how sick Yousef would be; afraid that he might die.

The people at the Erbprinz, the hotel in Germany, had become like family. They made us feel so at home and cared for. I missed that.

The next day, Yousef saw the hospital for the first time. It is an old building with so much character. We were welcomed to the ward upstairs. It felt very child-friendly, but I saw him in the waiting room looking out the window at the park across the way, watching the kids playing football.

"I can't wait to be playing football," he said.

"Yes, you will be soon," I said, believing with all my heart that it would be true one day.

We were greeted by the doctors, and we heard all about what was going to happen, how the weeks had been planned. Yousef's fifth round of chemo would begin right away, and his surgery would be five weeks later. It turned out that it had to be postponed since he wasn't well enough to keep on schedule. That night we returned home, and my dad's wife made Swedish meatballs. Yousef loved them. He ate with a very good appetite; he had not eaten meat for many months.

The next day, I had to go to the immigration office to sign us in. Yousef's immune system could not handle being around all the people who would be waiting there. He was scheduled to begin his treatment on Monday, and he could not afford to be exposed to all those germs. I went to immigration, and I was told the wait could be several hours. Yousef waiting in the car with my father. I waited for a long time and finally asked if it was possible that it could go quicker since I had a sick child sitting outside. It still took two hours. When my turn came, I asked the immigration official if he could come outside to the car to see my son. I knew it wasn't a normal request, so I was grateful when he kindly agreed. He understood Yousef couldn't risk getting sick. What a relief; now we were in "the system." I could finally stop holding my breath.

Sunday, we checked into the hospital, and the next morning Yousef got anti-nausea medication before the treatment even began. He still got sick, but less than it had been in Germany. Yousef even felt well enough to go down to the play area. He loved that there were things to do here in Sweden, unlike the hospital in Germany.

Chemo was very different in Sweden compared to what we were used to. The child receives anti-nausea meds before and during treatment to prevent illness. He is able to eat whatever food he liked and could tolerate. We were not expected to manage any part of the chemo at home; they kept Yousef in the hospital until he was well enough to be released. He didn't have to take antibiotics every single day, and it was a very child-friendly environment. I felt a great deal of support, which was a good thing because Yousef was quite sick. On Friday 12th June, I wrote in my diary,

When I look at Yousef, I want to cry because I feel so helpless. I can't make it easier for him! What else is possible? Today he woke up and his nose was bleeding, he had to have a hearing test, he was angry and depressed. In the afternoon his cast was looked at, and they were going to open it, and he screamed and was so afraid of having it cut off. He was so stressed that his shoulders went into spasm. They gave him something to calm him in order to check his cast, but he still wouldn't let them. They gave him painkillers for his neck and left him alone for the night."

We went through so much to get to Sweden, and it seemed like crossing such a hurdle, but here we were, still in the middle of chemo with more to come. Yousef would have to have his heart checked because of the strong chemo drugs. His red cell count was low, so he also had to be monitored in case he'd need a blood transfusion. The reality of the surgery was pressing on me as well. I would ask, "What will it take for Yousef's body to get strong?"

I would watch him sleep, sitting up folded over his leg. My sweet little boy was going through so much every day. He had all the side effects from the chemotherapy, but he was also still dealing with a broken leg and sores on his leg and the back of his foot from the cast. Whenever they had to open or fix his cast, he'd have to fast so they could give him anesthesia before the procedure. He was still traumatized from when his leg was cut the first time they opened his cast in Germany.

There were bright spots when my niece Johanna and her family came and visited us. It made Yousef so happy to see family and especially her little son Wilhelm, who was just over a year old at the time. He made Yousef laugh and smile from his heart.

The Astrid Lindgren Children's Hospital was very different from the Kinder Klinikum in Germany. Disney characters came through to entertain the children, volunteers offered activities such as music and arts and crafts. There was a common kitchen where we all could sit and eat. They had proper clowns who would come and entertain the families, to help everyone get through the difficult times. Even my father liked the clowns!

The children could collect beads from the Childhood Cancer Foundation. Each child would get a string and a hand-made bag to keep it in. They'd get a bead when they started treatment, and one for every injection, blood test, infusion, or other procedure they had to go through. Now, Yousef has this long strand.

"Look at how many injections I did," he said one day. It is actually a good memory, symbolic of all he has gone through.

We were in and out of the hospital all through June – Yousef was either in treatment or trying to get strong enough to continue. We had visits from my daughter and her friends, and we planned to see my sister in the north, but we wound up having to go back into the hospital instead. Yousef missed out on so many things – visits from friends and family that he just couldn't enjoy, a 4th of July party my oldest friend threw for him -- because he got a high fever. He was so upset to miss the barbeque that Cissi threw another one for him a week later when he felt better!

We finally went home on the 8th of July. My father and Runa were away, so we had the apartment to ourselves. Yousef was so happy, lying on the sofa bed with his sister Nathalie and her friend alongside him. These small memories of good times mean so much.

Yousef got stronger, and the time approached for his operation. We finally got to meet Dr. Otte in person. He was very straight with us, no BS. He is very confident, direct, but not unkind.

"Will I ever play football again? Yousef asked him.

"No," Dr. Otte said, "However, you could be a referee."

The doctor was very sure of himself, and I immediately had confidence in him, and I could tell Yousef did too. He told us about the preparation for the surgery, which would begin right away.

Starting five days before the operation, Yousef got injections to get his white blood cell count up. They had to build him up so he would be strong enough for the surgery. By this time, he was looking forward to it – he wanted to get the tumor out and to have his "new leg." The night before the operation, he wasn't nervous, but happy, and ready for the next day. In the morning, however, he woke up with a little anxiety in his eyes. In spite of that nervousness, he was excited to go.

## MINDFUL BREATHING

---

*Enlightenment comes when we realize happiness is a choice, sadness is a choice, anger is a choice, love is a choice.*

*— Brendan Burchard*

---

Somewhere in between the thing that hurts you and the way you react is a breath of time. It is all the time you need to change your outcome.

What you get handed today might stink. The situation you walk into might knock the wind right out of you. The conversation you have, the harsh words someone says because they are stressed – any of this and more – throws you for a loop. Then comes your choice. How to be, how to respond, how to stand in the midst of the hurricane and be unruffled.

Breathe. That small breath is stronger than the raging winds of the storm. Use it well.

*Breath is life. – William Atkinson*

## My Notes

# CHAPTER TEN

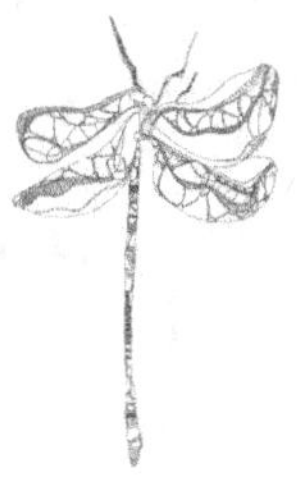

# I See The Future



At five minutes before 8:00 on 15 July, the day of the surgery, I still hadn't spoken with the surgeon. We were supposed to heading down to the operating room by this time. Finally, about a quarter after the hour, Dr. Otte came in. He seemed calm and answered a few questions I had. Finally, we were brought to the operating room. When we arrived, the whole team was already there waiting for Yousef.

Everything was very sterile, which is always important, but extremely so when it comes to an orthopedic operation. Yousef smiled when he saw the large, sparkling clean operating room. He was wheeled in and then moved over to the operation table, which had a special inflated, warm mattress. I was allowed to go in with him, but I was told to stay away from all the covered instruments.

I stood there and looked at the people busy preparing. I asked Yousef,

"So what are you going to dream about now? Imagine you are just going to sleep and you will have a dream, and when you wake up, I will be there next to you."

We spoke about the field we usually go to in our minds before we tell the Trouble Tree story. He mentioned his dog -- the German Shepherd he dreams of having one day.

The anesthesiologist came over, ready to put Yousef to sleep. Yousef seemed happy and totally calm. The medicine was put into his IV, and he was soon asleep.

"Sweet dreams, Yousef," I whispered.

I took a picture of him, sleeping. I kept my composure even though I felt emotional. I wanted to stay positive for him, so he wouldn't pick up negative feelings from me and get scared. Two nurses came over and walked me out. I understand that sometimes parents have a hard time leaving their child. They might faint, or make a scene.

"Thank you," they said to me.

"Why?"

"For making it easy for us. When a child is calm or just falls asleep, it is so much easier."

I left the hospital to walk on the grounds of the lovely Haga Parken – the national park right across from the hospital. It is the home of our royal Princess, and a place I had come to many times before. This is the park I used to walk in, and I did my normal route. The green all around me, the blue sky, it was warm, not hot – a pleasant day, with shady trees. I marveled at the Swedish summer, how different it was from the desert where I've lived for twenty-five years.

I appreciated the smell of the earth, the sound of the birds. It was very empty, early in the morning in the middle of the week. I looked over the field, remembering when I brought my girls here when they were small: 8 and 2 years old. It was December, and the park was full of snow. Twenty years ago, I had been in this same place sledding with my two small daughters – never imagining I'd be here today, waiting for my young son.

I walked quite a while, knowing the operation would take some time. I let myself feel the sun and warm breeze touch my face, allowing myself to breathe. I sat on a bench overlooking a slope that led down to a green field. It reminded me of the Trouble

Tree story Yousef asks for: a tranquil place, with trees to hang your worries. I was very worry-free this morning, in spite of the fact my child was in surgery. Nature is so healing. I just sat and listened to the birds and the leaves rattling in the wind. It was so calming. I had a feeling of trust and faith that everything would be alright.

On this same day in London, my younger daughter Nathalie was graduating from London College of Fashion, and I wasn't there with her. She had done really well and was an Honors student. I know it was hard for her. Not only was her mother not with her, but her little brother was having a huge operation to save his leg and his life. She was celebrating, and her brother was going through all this.

"Please, baby, go and enjoy your day," I said. I was relieved that her father was with her, so she wasn't alone, and she sent me pictures from her day.

I walked to the other side of the park and sat down on a bench and looked out. Across from me, down in the field, I saw a blond young man with his German Shepherd by his side.

Just before falling asleep, Yousef had spoken about a field where he was going to be with his German Shepherd – and here it was, that very scene. Like a snapshot of the future – a picture of Yousef as a young man, grown up and completely healed and well after all this, enjoying his life out in the sunshine with his beloved dog. I prayed it would be so.

The doctor called me around 11:00 am, two and a half hours after I'd left Yousef's side. I was a little surprised because I thought it might take the whole day. He told me to wait an hour or so, and then Yousef would be in recovery, and I would be able to see him.

When I returned to the hospital, I was shocked by what I saw. Yousef was so pale; he'd lost a lot of blood, and his leg was still bleeding. He had to stay in the recovery area for a couple of hours as the blood had to drain. He had a nerve block for his leg, otherwise, the pain would have been excruciating. You can imagine cutting and drilling into a bone. Even days later, they were giving him all sorts of medicines just to keep him out of pain. Yousef didn't do well; he was actually horrible on morphine – it affected his mood, his personality.

"Go away, I want to kill you!" he said to me one day in a voice I didn't even recognize.

For the next five days, I stayed next to him. On the 19th, his sister Salina came to visit with her husband, Liam, which meant I got a little bit of a break. Yousef wasn't feeling very well and wasn't very friendly toward his sister and brother-in-law. Liam helped a lot because he was patient and calm. Salina and Liam had rented an apartment, thinking that maybe, we could come and stay with them, but of course, it was too soon. Yousef wasn't doing well enough to leave the hospital.

Nathalie also came to see Yousef, and so did her dad, my ex-husband. Under the pain, Yousef did seem glad to have everyone there. I wish he could have enjoyed it more. For me, it meant I had a chance to go outside for a coffee by myself, to have a moment alone, away from Yousef's bedside. I also had the support of my daughters, which was so wonderful. They would listen and were very encouraging. My daughters would cook in the kitchen outside the ward, and Salina even baked pies and brought them to us. It was amazing to have home-cooked food after all this time.

I thought it was OK for me to leave Yousef for brief stretches of time, but, once when Nathalie was with him, he didn't feel comfortable telling her had to go to the bathroom. He wound up sitting in the mess until the next day, too embarrassed to tell anyone. The nurses helped us to take care of it, and I told him not to be ashamed. I realized I couldn't take more than a short time away from him.

Immediately after the surgery, Yousef was supposed to start moving his leg. He couldn't put any pressure on it yet, but the nurses and physiotherapists would come and try to begin exercising it to help the healing. They couldn't let it drop or lower it all the way to the floor yet. Yousef would scream no matter how careful they were or how slowly they moved him.

It was ten days after the surgery before Yousef moved to a wheelchair and the therapists slowly started to lower his leg to the floor. He looked so weak and yellow. It would still be some time before he could stand, but this was a big step. Once he was in the wheelchair, we could take him outside. One day we all played outside, and even Yousef had fun and enjoyed some ice cream. On other days, he wasn't doing well at all. On the Sunday before Salina and Liam were to leave, we planned to have big celebration brunch in the park where I'd walked the day of the surgery. We were all looking forward to it so much, but Yousef didn't feel well enough to go, and I didn't want to leave him.

Salina and Liam spoiled us while they were there. They bought us an espresso machine and a TV and told us that we would have our own home soon. It was sad to see them go. Right after they left, Yousef moved to Q84, the oncology floor, to prepare for his next round of chemo. It was only 11 days after his operation. I wondered how he would manage it.

I know we have a choice about how to feel, even when things are difficult. I kept telling myself that I can choose to be happy during this difficult time. It was important to keep asking the question, 'What can I do to make it better?' I chose to take it one moment at a time and to be the best possible mother to Yousef I could be, in each moment. In order to do that, I had to be as clear as I could about my own thoughts and feelings.

We were alone together again. We had a routine: I'd make breakfast, we'd watch a couple of TV shows in the morning, sitting together in the bed. Then he'd go to physiotherapy. In the beginning, he would scream like crazy, but it got better over time. He started to enjoy arts and crafts, and it kept him busy. He started to crave all sorts of food because he could have whatever he wanted, and his appetite was back. He asked for cake, which he loves. I was glad I could cook for him in the kitchen on Q84.

At the "Lekterapin," the activity center, the children are free to express themselves in so many ways, and now that Yousef was feeling better, he could enjoy it. The people who work there are all truly wonderful, so caring and giving. They make the hospital stay a little easier for the children, siblings, and parents.

At Astrid Lindgren, they've also thought of the children who can't go down to the Lekterapin because they're having chemo. They have a team called "Pysselbyrån" (Arts & Crafts) who would come around to us. I used to look forward to them because they came smiling, with themes and activities for adults and children alike. They were a distraction from the routine that you learn to accept as the new reality. Arts and crafts, play, and music therapy – they all help to give your child (and you) a break. Maybe it also helps everyone to emotionally process what's going on.

On the 31st of July, Yousef stood up for the first time. He had tears streaming down his cheeks. He was elated, screaming from pain and excitement. I have a picture from that day. This moment was a confirmation to him that he would be able to use his leg again. It had been 5 months and 7 days since he had last stood. When he was recently asked what it felt like to be able to stand up again on his own two legs, all he said was,

"Amazing."

How does it get any better than that?

After physio that day, we went upstairs to the ward, and he wanted to sit in the living room! Then on his own, he wheeled himself to the examination room where his favorite nurse, Christopher, gave him his injection and medicines. Christopher told me afterward that he took them easily.

Yousef came back out to the living room to do some activity as "pyssel byrån," (arts and crafts,) had come. He made a beautiful painting. Then we left the hospital and came home. That night, before falling asleep, he read a whole chapter in his new book, <u>The Mystery of the Griefer's Mark</u>- a Mine Craft book.

Wow what a day, I thought. I was so happy for him. What if tomorrow could be an even better day? What else is possible?

At the end of July, things were looking much better. I was excited to write my diary entry for Thursday 30 July 2015,

What a day today has been! This morning, Yousef woke up in a really good mood. He started writing today's schedule then had his breakfast. At 9.30 am he had his heart test, which was good. Then he came back to the room and slept for over an hour.

At 1:00 pm we had an appointment with the Physio. There, Yousef played the Wii game "Mario Kart " while one of the Physiotherapist lowered his leg. It was down on the floor for 10 minutes! Afterward, he moved over to the barre where he was able to stand up, holding on while they managed to lower his leg all the way down to the floor. He stood on both legs for 5 minutes!

Such simple things, and so amazing!

I've written a bit about getting support, and I really believe having people you can rely on is so important. There were psychologists we could have spoken to, and I am sure they are very useful to some people. When we were in Germany, a psychologist came to see Yousef, but she had an approach that didn't work. Yousef refused to speak with her every time she came. When we got to Sweden, the psychologist had a different approach, and she accepted that Yousef didn't want to talk. Instead, Yousef was offered music therapy, and he later met Andreas in the "Lekterapin." He and Andreas connected – and he taught Yousef to create his own music.

There was also a woman who made films with the children, and Yousef loved that. They used an app on the iPad, and Yousef used his own Legos, which are his favorite toys. When I watched him, I thought even if he has missed almost a year of school, he's learned so many other things this year.

---

*Worry pretends to be necessary, but serves no purpose."*

*- Eckhardt Tolle*

---

Sometimes, our mind runs away with us. Off we go, and now, we aren't free, we are captive. We aren't able to be present with others. We don't have space in our hearts for care or listening. Our minds are racing, and it takes up all the room in our hearts that we need for other things. Now is not the time to allow worry to drag us away. Let worry go on its way, alone. Watch it, like a cloud slips from your view…like a wave recedes back into the ocean.

Whenever you are getting carried away with worry, close your eyes for a moment.

Imagine you are holding a piece of chalk in your hand.

See a chalkboard in front of you.

Begin writing numbers down, as if you are making a list.

1.

2.

3.

etc.

Now, see yourself writing down the first thing that is bothering you – the worst thing. Condense it down to a few words, or maybe just one word.

Now, watch your other hand as it picks up an eraser or a rag. Erase the worry. Go over each letter until there isn't a trace to be seen of the words you've written about your worry or concern.

When the worry has been entirely wiped away, go on to number 2. In your mind's eye, see yourself write the next concern. Again, condense it to just a few words. Now, pick up the eraser and wipe it completely away.

Do this for each and every worry you have: letting your mind acknowledge and then erase and release them.

You can do this exercise to help you relax or to fall asleep at night, too. It comes from a hypnosis technique.

To use it for that purpose, see yourself writing numbers from 10 down to 1, erasing them as you go.

For example:

In your mind's eye, see your hand writing the number "10."

Then, see your hand erasing the number "10" completely.

Watch your hand writing number "9." Imagine erasing "9", and so on.

## My Notes

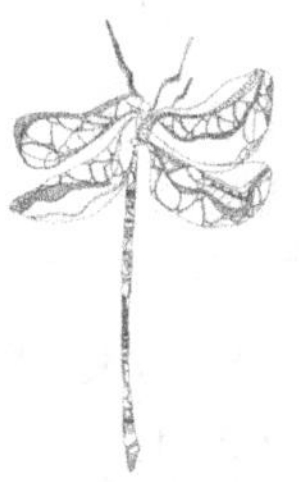

# Now I Have More Time

---

*You will never have this day with your children again. Tomorrow they will be a little older than they were today. This day is a gift."*

*– Sutton Coldfield*

---

One day, Yousef asked me, ""How do you get cancer?"

"I don't know. Let's ask the doctor," I said.

So when he came up from his next Physio appointment, he did. It was a doctor he said he didn't like just a few days before. I don't know if he was satisfied with her answer.

"No one knows for sure," she said.

"Can you get more cancers?" he asked.

"Sadly, yes," she said.

The doctor told Yousef she was very happy he was asking questions, she said he could ask anytime, through me, or directly.

It was natural for him to wonder about it for himself, but he had also just seen his friend Justin experience a recurrence of leukemia. Justin had been doing well after treatment, and just as everyone thought he was in the clear, he got sick again.

As I write this, Justin is recovering from having a bone marrow transplant. As soon as he is well enough for visitors, Yousef wants to go and see him.

Yousef has seen and experienced too much for his years. He also knows that his grandmother is dying of cancer. There is a lot of illness around him. I would love him never to have to wonder about getting sick again or dying prematurely. But, he is reminded of his condition all the time, and he will be checked and treated for years to come. I tell him that no one is promised a certain number of years – at any moment, any one of us might die from cancer or something else. It's a lesson that many adults don't even understand, and my nine-year-old was confronted with it every day. As for me, I feel blessed that, now, I have more time with Yousef. Anything could happen to anyone, any day. I am now with him, and I appreciate every moment.

Astrid Lindgren Children's Hospital had many things to keep our spirits up, and not just for the patients and parents. There was a woman who ran activities for the young siblings of the patients because they need attention, too. She baked each morning for all of us. We'd wake up to the good smell of vanilla and cinnamon. One day, there was a band on the oncology floor – and of course, there were clowns! It was such a healing environment, very positive and child-friendly. When we were there, it felt very supportive, very good.

Going home to my father's apartment, however, was another story. Just getting into the apartment was a challenge. They live up a flight of stairs, and I would have to carry Yousef up, then go back down and carry up the wheelchair. I don't know where I got the strength from – it's incredible how you can do anything when you just focus on it.

Yousef used to hug me and say, "I love you, Mamma! Thank you for taking care of me!"

That gave me even more strength. Only later did a driver tell me there was a stair climber in some of the wheelchair taxis.

"No one mentioned it to you?" he asked.

"No, I didn't know you could even ask for such a thing."

My father apologized that he couldn't help more. Living at his apartment was a challenge in other ways. He and Runa were set in their ways, and I felt we were in their way, interrupting their routine. I appreciated their support and was grateful when my father tried to joke with Yousef, even if he was surly in his reply sometimes because he wasn't feeling well.

Things were complicated in more ways than that. When Yousef started school in September, he was still under treatment. Imagine having to start a new school (not just a new school *year*) sick from chemo and still recovering from surgery! Plus, we had just moved into our own apartment. Yousef could now stand on his crutches, but he became exhausted if he had to walk too far or stand for too long. He was happy that day.

Yousef found that school in Sweden is different from Dubai. Here, students have hot lunch and breakfast and fruit during the day for snacks. Yousef stays after school for junior club where he takes part in different activities such as "Home Ec." He has a snack and an after-school program called "Research and Development," which is supervised time to do homework. In Dubai, you bring your own lunch, pay for extracurricular activities, and there is no time after school to do your homework with supervision! But Yousef had to learn to deal with how his peers would react to him. I don't know what makes kids so cruel sometimes, but Yousef, sadly, had to deal with bullying in his new school, right alongside everything else.

Sometimes, I watch Yousef hopping around on his leg, and I am amazed by how well he has adjusted and how happy he is most of the time. Salina has reflected on how Yousef is now: open, and able to communicate easily with me. He might be moody, but he is getting into his teen years, so it might be perfectly normal, not related at all to after-effects of treatment or his physical condition – just puberty!

For Yousef, the whole experience was about more than the illness, treatment, or even the surgery. There was the shock of breaking his leg during his favorite activity at school and having to accept that he would never play football again. Then he was torn away from his childhood home and country, his school, and his friends. He was separated from his father, brother, and sisters. He had to live in Germany - a foreign country with a different language then move again for surgery, which was terrifying all by itself. – He had visited my family in Sweden before but had never lived there. I can't tell you how hard it was adjusting to the ways of a different hospital where the routines and attitude were so different from the Kinder Klinikum in Germany.

You don't realize that you enter a culture – a way to practice medicine that is unique to that hospital. Leaving it means you take your disease, at whatever stage, and you enter a whole new culture and have to learn how it works. You miss some of the things from the last place – even though you'd never choose in a million years to be in either one.

Yousef is still adjusting to the after-effects of his surgery and the new reality of his body now. That's a lot for a little boy. Recently, he wrote an essay for school. The actual assignment was to imagine having to leave your home because of war – becoming a refugee, forced to leave your friends and family because of violence. But Yousef wrote it from his personal experience.

"I don't have to imagine war," he said, "I had to leave my home and friends and school."

I agreed. Look at the language we use about cancer: we fight it, or it's called a battle for your life, and we want to "beat it." Yousef didn't have to imagine being a refugee because of a war.

## Awareness

---

If you could be calm and centered whenever you had to explain something to your child, or when you ask some questions of the doctor, how would that help?

If you could become mindful and aware of something soothing or beautiful in your surroundings once (or more) per day- what might be different?

<u>A Practice to Try:</u>

Become conscious of the room you are in. Locate something that looks beautiful or attractive to you. Maybe you can look at a window, at trees, or the sky.

Or, find something that gives you a sense of love or peace.

Become aware of the beauty, love, or peace. Focus on it.

Breathe.

Say, "And now I am fully here. Not in the future or the past. Right here and right now. Hear clearly. I ask for what I need, right now, in this moment."

Breathe.

My Notes

# CHAPTER TWELVE

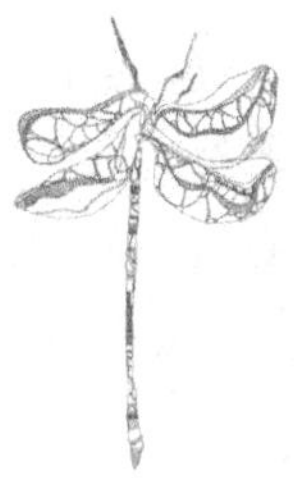

# Inspiring Friends



*"I never met a bitter person who was thankful. Or a thankful person who was bitter."*

— *Nick Vujicic*

We are never the same after cancer. Not as individuals, or as a family. Plenty of times, cancer doesn't kill the patient, but it can definitely kill marriages, cause rifts in families, and breaks between friends. Cancer shows us how fear brings out the worst in people. For example, at school Yousef experienced bullying – with one child threatening to kick him in the leg; even telling him, "I hope you get the cancer back!" What makes a child say something like that? It didn't seem there was anything personal between them, no animosity, no fight. But kids can be so cruel – and I think it was out of fear. Yousef walked a little differently, and he started school in a wheelchair, and it made him the target of a bully. And we all know bullies are children (and adults) who have been picked on and feel inadequate themselves.

Cancer can open our eyes, too. We see the job, or the life we had wasn't worth all the lifetime we were devoting to it. We realize: nobody is promised tomorrow, and now is the time to live the life we dreamed of. Sometimes that means leaving jobs or lifestyles or relationships. It can mean we finally get the courage to pursue our dreams. Cancer changes us and everything around us, and sometimes, if we are intentional about it, it can change our lives for the better. We figure out that now is the time to appreciate the people we love and do and say what is in our hearts.

"What would you like people to know about what you've been through?" I asked Yousef recently.

"How it is to sit in bed all day long with nothing to do – so people know that there are people in the world who can't do anything but sit and wait," Yousef said. He learned empathy, and he wanted to teach that to others.

"People will know what I've been through, and what others are going through," he said.

My friend Shaikha lost her arm to cancer when she was only two. Shaikha is an inspiration. She says people who stare or judge her are "silly." She knows it is a prejudice that comes from fear. She says, yes, she is different, meaning unique, unlike the ordinary rest of the world. She is a living example of self-acceptance and courage. I asked her what she would tell a child and his or her parents about the lasting effects of cancer, particularly when their bodies look or work differently afterward.

**Me: You were very young when you lost your arm, but it impacted the rest of your life in ways that most of us cannot imagine. What would you like us to know about you?**

- At the beginning, I was always upset about being different from other kids. I was not accepted by the children around me, and they used to tease me about my prosthetic arm. I realized that wearing it does not add anything to me. It just makes people think that I look like them. Eventually, I decided to step up and face my life without wearing it.

**What would you tell a child who worries that they will be "different" after their illness?**

- I'd tell them don't feel "different," feel special because you are special and unique.

Most of the people out there are alike, yet God has chosen us to look unique and special.

**What encouragement or words of wisdom would you give to parents about how to cope with the physical changes their child might experience?**

- Stay strong. Being upset about something that took place will not change the fact of the disease, or (in my case) the limb the child lost. Feeling sorry or looking at him with pity will not make him stronger. The damage is done. Work together to make the child more confident, let him be independent, let him try and fail. The more he tries, the better he will be. When kids in school make fun of the child, teach him how to respond and act. Don't feel sorry, or go down to the school to handle it for him. That makes him feel weaker. Teach him to survive without you. By doing too much for the child, he will never learn he can do it himself, which is not right in my opinion. They need to learn the hard way to succeed in their life. They need to make the child proud of how he looks and who he is. Do not look at your child with pity all the time.

**What did your own parents do RIGHT? What would you have preferred they do differently?**

- My parents, God bless them, were the exact opposite. My dad was over-protective and always feels sorry for me and thinks that I need help in every single thing I do. My mum made me not feel any different in anything. She never treated me differently even when I could not handle things like tying my hair, carrying things, drawing lines on the notebook. However, she wasn't mean, she just made me learn how to handle things on my own and to figure out a way to do things without anyone's help. It takes a brave mum to do that for her child, especially after all the medical treatments the child has gone through. But, here I am standing in front of the world proud of who I am, where I am, and how I look. A huge "thank you" goes to my mother who suffered by raising me to make me who I am now.

**What would you say to a child, to encourage, console or inspire?**

- Love yourself for who you are. Be proud of how you look. Feel that you're special. YOU ARE UNIQUE. Move on and try to inspire the world with what you can do. Listen, pick and choose what you hear from people. Turn the sentences that have a negative impact on you into a positive sentence. Remember, in spite of someone's silly words: YOU ARE UNIQUE.

**You are so inspirational! What have people said to you about your attitude, belief, abilities?**

- Believe it or not, I am very happy with the way I look and never want to wear a prosthetic. All it does is please people's eyes. I am here the way I am. I have accepted myself and love the way I look. I am living my life better than any normal person. Accept yourself, love yourself, believe in your capabilities. Disability is not when you have a missing limb, it's when you stop and limit yourself.

**I understand not everyone has been kind to you. How do you handle their reactions? What would you say to a parent, or a child, who might find themselves facing some harsh or bullying experiences as a result of their illness?**

- I am who I am. I have accepted how I look, now the world has to accept me. I give a huge smile, and I think twice before reacting. In the beginning, it's the parents who have to help the child accept what happened to them. The parent should make the child feel confident, even when people stare or point at them. If a parent is over-protective, the child is weaker in personality. Do speak to the child every now and then. Show him movies, real stories where people deal with disabilities or illness, so he can see it happens to others in the world. It will help the child develop the ability to build more confidence in themselves.

**What have you learned about life, about others, and about yourself as a result of your different-ability?**

- I have learned that life is not easy, but you can handle it with the right perspective. I learned that, in general, people will underestimate you regardless of your disability. That is human nature. But, YOU ARE THE SPECIAL ONE. You change the world by being yourself and doing all you are able to do. That will teach other people how to see you – you will show them what "different" means.

Sometimes I watch Yousef hopping around on his leg, and I am amazed by how well- adjusted and happy he is most of the time. He might get moody, but he is getting into his teen years, so it might be perfectly normal, not related at all to after-effects of treatment or his physical condition.

When we were in Germany, I heard about a man called Nicholas Vujicic, an Australian born with Tetra-Amelia Syndrome, a rare disorder characterized by the absence of arms and legs. Today, Nick is a motivational speaker and author of seven books. He writes about life, love, and self-acceptance. He writes about family, productivity, work, and the power of faith and standing strong. Despite suffering from bullying and struggling mentally and physically, he didn't give up.

I showed Yousef some of his YouTube videos. He was inspired how Nick was able to move without any legs and arms. And how he didn't give up. Yousef said,

"He inspired me by how he can go every day, and he makes jokes about himself, and he's always happy. He can do a lot of stuff."

I asked him what he learned from Nick, and he said,

"Try to be happy all the time."

Last year in October, Nick came to Stockholm. Yousef and I went to hear him speak, and we got a chance to meet him. It was an amazing experience for Yousef. Once again, he was shown that you can always do things if you believe you can, and it's okay if you don't make it right, you just try again. I have a picture of Yousef hugging Nick, which I just love. Nick says,

"... for every disability you have, you are blessed with more than enough abilities to overcome your challenges."

No, Nick couldn't hug Yousef back with his arms, but his attitude and what he taught Yousef was even better, more powerful, more lasting. He had the ability to more than overcome his challenges, and so does Yousef.

## My Notes

# CHAPTER THIRTEEN

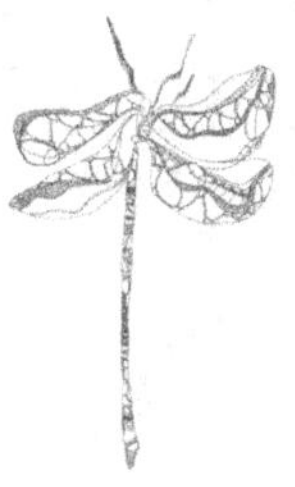

# Fear Is a Dragon

---

*"It is impossible to control your thoughts. They happen at the speed of light. But…the one thing you do have control over is how you react to the thought you just had."*

*– Trevor Blake*

---

Yousef finished chemo at the end of November. On the day he was discharged, the doctor gave me all the paperwork and instructions for follow-ups. I had no idea what to expect.

"Oh my God!"

He handed me the plan for ten years' worth of follow-ups that would include check-ups every six weeks in the first year, then every three months in the second. He'd need blood work, chest X-rays, and X-rays of his leg. In addition, any time we planned to travel, he'd need a check-up first. All of this is just for the cancer, not the leg. For that, we have a whole different protocol!

Yousef's birthday is December 2nd, and his wish was to spend it back home in Dubai. We planned to go, but I knew we probably wouldn't be able to make it in time for his birthday. So I arranged for Salina, Liam, Jill, Ramsey, and Nathalie all to come home (to Sweden) that weekend to surprise him. He'd wanted that too: for everyone to be there for his birthday. When the doorbell rang, and they were all there, he couldn't believe his eyes!

We went to the museum together, Yousef in the wheelchair. He really enjoyed it. Then we had a combined party to celebrate both finishing his treatment and his birthday. While I'd planned the weekend, I'd been counting the days, thinking that he could very well be in the hospital, sick from the after-effects of his last round of chemo. Normally, this would have been the week when he'd be very weak and prone to complications. Yousef got lucky. He never had to go back into the hospital again. Yousef had learned that many times I couldn't keep promises because things out of our control would come up. We had an understanding. We would plan and go forward as if things would work out, but we would accept it if something happened to change our plans. He never questioned me.

We did get to Dubai later in December, although, right up to the last day I wasn't sure he'd be well enough to fly. The trip to Dubai was very emotional. Yousef was in compression socks for the plane and still in his difficult-to-manage wheelchair, and we were returning for the first time in nearly a year to where this journey had begun. We were not the same people, but he'd looked forward to it so much, and it was great for him to be there.

Salina had arranged a picnic at the beach, and our family and friends came. It was still a little cool in Dubai, but Yousef loved being in the sand. Dubai isn't as wheelchair-friendly as other parts of the world, so he had to move around more on his crutches, which was a boost for him – it gave him some independence. He had to use his leg a bit more, and he started believing in himself and in his leg. He saw that it was OK to use it. He knew there were stairs to get into our building before the elevator. We could carry him, but he practiced in order to do it by himself. He was able to visit his old school, and he stayed with his friends for a whole day. He still stays in touch with them through Skype and Minecraft. It seems those boys are in my house all the time through that technology.

We spent the New Year in Dubai and came back to Sweden in the middle of January. He'd missed a bit of school, but I thought that was alright under the circumstances, although, the school isn't always so happy when I keep him out for travel or whatever. We both feel school and education are important, but so is enjoying life, experiencing new things, and seeing family and friends. Cancer puts everything into perspective.

Yousef realizes he can't go back to Dubai to live, but the trip was reassuring. It's only a six-hour flight away. He might not be living there, but he can visit. Recently I asked him whether he wanted to go and live in Dubai again.

"No, I want to live in Sweden."

I don't know why he prefers it; maybe he realizes they don't have the treatment options for cancer in Dubai. His father has also told him that the doctors are better in Sweden. The hospital is familiar, and they take good care of him. He knows and trusts his surgeon. Maybe he feels safe here.

I know he thinks about things that he doesn't talk about. His friend Justin almost died of leukemia. He started his chemo much earlier than Yousef. He went through so much - he was in a coma for six weeks. When Justin finished up his treatment, everyone thought he was going to be fine. When he got sick again, it was such a shock to Yousef, and he was so upset. Justin became really depressed; he didn't want to live and fight anymore.

Justin's mother is afraid.

"What will it take for you to let that go?" I asked her.

"I am afraid to believe it's going to be OK," she said.

Of course, Yousef is aware of all this, but he doesn't talk about it.

When we came back from Dubai this year in January, my step-mother was back in hospital with cancer. We knew she was dying. That was when Yousef started asking whether you can get cancer again. I knew I had to be careful talking to him, not to upset him and add to his concerns.

Yousef is keeping his attitude up; he's not depressed, but no one knows what Methotrexate, one of his main chemo drug, does to the mind. It might cause anxiety or depression. They do a lot of follow-up on that, asking about his moods, thoughts, and effect. I asked the psychologist recently about some of his moodiness.

"Is it the Methotrexate or the after-effects of chemo in general – or is it puberty?!"

Nobody seems to know for sure. I'm going to look at him as a budding teenager and let it be.

When we were in Germany, and they first released Yousef to me between treatments, they sent me home with shots and pills and a strict schedule to follow to manage his nausea and counteract the chemo. They released us with stern warnings to watch his diet and look out for dangerous side effects. They sent me off all by myself, with a boy who was so sick. It was terrifying. I had a milder form of that same feeling when they signed us out of Q84 at Astrid Lindgren for the last time. I felt very much on my own. I am sure other patients and family members feel that way.

There is a study in Canada where they followed families after their children were released from cancer treatment. The effects on a family can be devastating, and the feeling of being completely alone once they are discharged from the hospital or from treatment is frightening and common. The study found that if the family is followed by a coach, after six months, the children and the whole family are doing much better than families without one. Coaching improves the outcome of long-term recovery and the health of the family system.

In my opinion, coaching can, at times, be more effective to deal with more things than psychotherapy. Psychologists focus on analyzing the source of fear, and they focus on the past. Coaching focuses on the now and on the future. It is positive and forward-looking. I'd much rather ask, "What do we do now? Here we are, a family, we are different now. We have a child who has gone through this difficult thing – and now, what?"

I believe you don't go into the fear. Instead, you look at the possibilities. That is what coaching does. It's like being confronted with a monster, say, a dragon. As a coach, I would say, "See your dragon (fear), and ask what can I do with that?"

Likewise, I don't focus on what Yousef can't do but what he CAN do. His surgeon, Dr. Otte has the same approach. When Yousef told him he wanted to play football, Dr. Otte said,

"What if you could be the referee?"

Our minds will limit everything unless we focus differently. There is life after cancer, and what you must focus on is *life*. I encourage Yousef to look at what he <u>will</u> be able to do – bicycle, or swim -- rather than what he cannot. I think about what happens to children after they are released from their treatment and rehabilitation. They don't have coaches; and through the long months of illness and debilitating chemo, they learn about limitation instead of possibility. What would it take to turn that around?

Three hundred kids each year used to be diagnosed with cancer in Sweden, and today that number has risen to 350 – every year. The population here is small, so that is a really big number. Survival rates are improving, and in the future, will get even better, but cancer isn't going away. The world isn't getting less toxic. How will we help those children to adjust to their new reality and make the most of everything they have experienced and learned?

## Butterfly Hug

**What might be possible if your body and mind were brought into alignment and peace, physiologically?** This practice is called bilateral stimulation. It is said to balance the mind and body and to reduce anxiety. Here is how to do it:

Cross your arms over your chest as if you are hugging yourself. Put your hands on opposite biceps, like this:

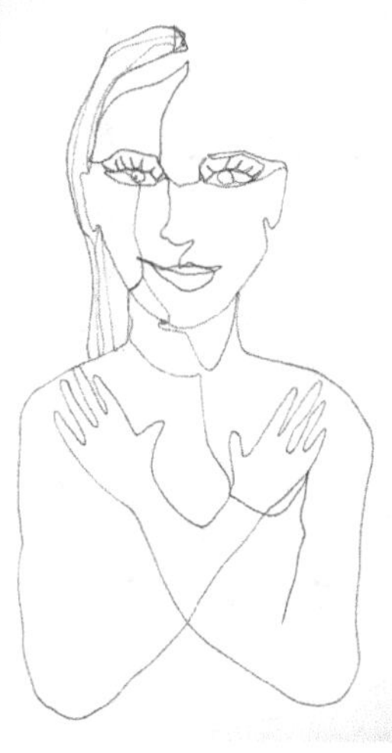

Slowly and gently tap, first one hand, then the other, on your arm.

Do this while you breathe in and out five times. Deep slow breaths.

*You can teach your child to do the Butterfly Hug as well. It will give him or her a way to self-soothe whenever they need to.*

## AMANDA'S STORY

I interviewed Amanda Eriksson, who was a first-time mother when her three-month-old daughter was diagnosed with cancer. I've translated their story from Swedish.

**Helene: As a young new mother, hearing your baby is sick is just devastating. Can you give us just a couple of sentences that tell our readers what happened to your family? (What was the diagnosis, how did you find out your daughter was sick, what the treatment was?)**

Estelle was born in September 2014. Around Christmas time, when she was 3 months old, she started getting a cold and had a fever on and off through January and February. She also had a severe cough and developed croup. We were in and out of the emergency room. She had bacteria in the urine all the time, but the doctors blamed it on the bacteria in the diaper. In the end, now early March, the nurse at our pediatric clinic sent us to get an ultrasound to see whether the bacteria had spread to the kidneys. They found a tumor larger than a tennis ball on Estelle's left kidney. When the doctor called and said they'd found something, I didn't know how serious it was. But two hours later, we were at the children's oncology ward, and that same evening they began chemotherapy. In the following ten months, Estelle went through surgery, radiation, and frequent chemotherapy treatments. She had clear cell sarcoma, a rare kidney tumor.

**What did you do to try to mother your infant in normal ways? For example, I know you breastfed through chemo. Tell us about that. What else?**

I breastfed Estelle throughout the treatment and continued even a few months afterward. I am so grateful that I had the opportunity to do this, and it made it easier for all needle sticks and check-ups. The best thing was to have my beloved daughter next to me and feel her breath and heart beating against me. The two of us became one and created the vital ties to heal each other's hearts.

We were living under very difficult circumstances and mostly isolated from other children and families, but the staff at the oncology ward Q84 were amazing, Pysselbyrån (Arts & Crafts) and Lekterapin (play-therapy center) were incredibly important for us. Even music became important. We brought Estelle's children songs with us, ones we've played since she was born. I remember how we danced every day in the room or in the kitchen of the ward. We sang a lot, laughed and hugged. We were always together, the three of us, we were and still are the strongest when we're together!

**What was important for your self-care?**

I lost myself completely during Estelle's treatment. I did not leave her for a second, even when I would take a shower, I took her into the bathroom. If we had anything to buy, my partner Calle had to go. Sometimes I forced myself to go out for a walk to get fresh air and leave the hospital walls. Haga Parken was an oasis. I walked around and cried and let everything go, and then filled myself with a new energy that gave me new strength and courage, I was recharged. I even wrote a diary, and it was liberating to get out all the feelings and experiences. And even now, in hindsight, it is nice to revisit.

**Where did your support come from?**

My beloved Calle, Estelle's father. We were each other's best **friends in** life's worst moments. As well as my family, some friends, and of course, all the fantastic hospital staff.

**How are you a different parent than you might have been otherwise?**

I wake up every day and thank the higher powers that Estelle is next to me. I am present in a totally different way, I do not stress and worry about the little things. I give Estelle all my time. I dare to say NO to things I do not want to do or feel I don't have the strength for. I am staying with my family's energy and mine.

**Tell us how your daughter is now (people will want to read it for encouragement!)**

Today, Estelle is 3 years old and is doing well. She is the world's most wonderful, empathetic, and precocious girl! She feels much wiser - beyond her 3 years, and she makes my heartbeat flip every day. Her love gets my feet to take off with ease. With her, everything is possible!

**You were a young, first-time mum when your child got sick. Probably, lots of your expectations of your baby's early months went out the window. Can you say anything about that?**

I grieved for a long time, and still do today, that all parental leave (in Sweden the maternal/paternal leave is 18 months) was used to struggle for our daughter's life. Other mothers met at the open pre-school, had coffee in the park, traveled, fed their children with porridge and purees, struggling with sleepless nights, etc. We were isolated in a room at the children's cancer ward. It felt like we were struggling between life and death, not knowing which way we would fall. It felt like my heart had a thousand holes that constantly oozed blood. But while everything was sad and incredibly heavy, we had the world's finest days according to our conditions. Every day with Estelle felt like the most beautiful, and it is nice to look back on.

**Tell me anything else you think might be important.**

I would like to highlight the importance of family and friends' support. Dare to contact/call, dare to show that you care and are thinking of the family. Just a text message every now and then, or come by with a lunch box. Why not send a postcard to the department? Do not be afraid to interfere, but expect no answer. Do not ever stop showing your concern!

Hugs,
Amanda

*My Notes*

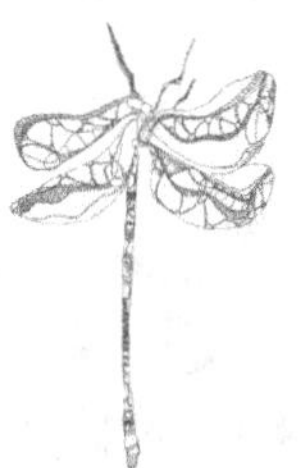

# CHAPTER FOURTEEN

# What Are We Going To Do With It?

---

*"If I fail, I try again, and again, and again. If YOU fail, are you going to try again? The human spirit can handle much worse than we realize. It matters HOW you are going to FINISH. Are you going to finish strong?"*

*– Nick Vujicic*

---

We are now in the long, watchful state of recovery. We are past the chemo, but still dealing with the possibility of after-effects *from* chemo. Yousef's treatments are over, but he still has frequent check-ups, tests, and scans to see that the cancer stays away. We are past surgery, but we still have to worry about Yousef's leg, which will never grow on its own. It can only be lengthened so far mechanically -- and then what? We will face that when the time comes.

The life we have now has been shaped by our cancer experience. Whatever adjustments we make every day are just a part of who we are and what we do now. Whatever new strength, awareness, and determination come from that place too. We are stronger than when the cancer interrupted our life because now we look at everything differently.

Like us, you can get through and see your life differently. You don't need to be fearful, bitter or broken. I promise, you have the power to choose how to handle whatever the diagnosis brings, and you *can* guide your child through this. It won't be easy, but you have everything you need to handle it. And if you don't feel so strong all the time, then do not hesitate for a moment to ask for the help you need.

I have always been a positive person, and throughout this whole ordeal, I decided crying wouldn't help anyone. I was determined to be the best possible support for my son. Of course, there were times I did cry, but not in front of Yousef. There were times when I was so afraid, confused, and frustrated – even with my child, who would sometimes resist the medicines or injections I would have to give him. In those raw times, I knew I had to step away so that I could be a help and support to him and not let my emotions run away with me.

I'm sure I didn't do everything right. Neither will you. There is so much parents need to know in order to talk to a child about scary and complicated diagnoses and protocols. You will hear A LOT of information in a short period of time – too much to understand. You will have a hundred questions and not be clear on the answers. You need to weed all that out to make decisions and then tell your child what he or she needs to know. It's OK to make mistakes, to feel like you don't know what you are doing. You can and will figure it out. Be gentle with yourself. One of the physiotherapists at Astrid Lindgren wrote about how important parental support is – and how strong the kids are!

Emilie wrote,

"Working…with children with cancer is difficult but also incredibly rewarding. It is a complex disease, and what is good to do one day may not work at all the day after depending on how the children are doing…the progress is not linear. It is because of the highs and the lows that the child needs more responsiveness from parents and caregivers. But, what I am struck by constantly is how strong the little superheroes are, and how they often will find their own strategies to solve the challenges that we adults never thought about!"

My own little superhero did better than me some days! He handled so much with such courage – and he still does. Someone asked him, "What would you tell another kid who had to go through what you did?"

"I would say, there are days that are really tough and shitty, but there are days that are really fun. Enjoy the time you have and don't think about the negative."

Maybe that sounds more profound coming from him than me! But, I've found there is always something good to notice, even though you might have to look quite hard to find it some days.

Early on in all of this, I decided I would try to grow from what we were going through. It might sound crazy considering how much fear and uncertainty there was. But, we are all tested sometimes, and in the test, is the chance to dig deep inside yourself and grow – to decide who you are. What might you discover about yourself or your child?

What we think about is so important, and yet, so many thoughts are anxious reactions to what goes on around us. Yes, bad things happen, our kids get sick. And, the question is, what are we going to do with it?

I also decided to "pay it forward," and that's what this book is about. I hope to make donations from its proceeds, and I want to help other families going through the same thing we did. This book is not necessarily just for parents, but other people dealing with cancer, or the problems of illness, the medical system, or coping with life and death issues. Yousef is already asking about my next book, too!

I rely on questions – they are the foundation of my life. Questions empower us, and thinking we have all the answers disempowers. That's when we stop looking for miracles and opportunities. Being in the question, never claiming to know the answer, that's where the possibilities are.

A question can change the energy of any situation you find yourself in. Being willing to continually ask will open the door to a whole different life. Whenever something challenged me, I would ask, "What else is possible now?" As I tried my best to get through the past three years, I must have asked it a thousand times, for a thousand different reasons.

Thoughts are reactions to what goes on around us. I've learned not to believe the first thought, but to ask a question and see if the thought can be changed to something positive. Yousef seems to have learned that, too!

I am grateful - I am sure that sounds strange to some people. But through this experience, I learned to take nothing for granted and to live in the NOW. We could be taken away from each other at any moment, so we have to be there for each other and for ourselves. I have the gift of more time with Yousef. Who knows how long any of us have with our children? Don't wait for someone to get sick to begin to appreciate the time. Don't wait for <u>anything.</u>

I would tell a parent going through what I went through to remember all of your children need you, even as you have to devote yourself to the one who is sick. I had to be there for all my children, and so will you. During this time, my eldest daughter had just gotten married, and my younger daughter was finishing University. My older son was applying to go to University. They all needed my support, too. I am proud of all of them – how they were there for their brother, and each contributed what he or she could.

I am the mother of four. I've always put everyone else before me. I've learned how important it is to take care of myself, now. I think about the salt baths I took in Germany, in the privacy of my hotel room. They were more than a retreat – they were healing, a chance to stop thinking, to switch off. Through our time in hospitals, I didn't always have this luxury, but I'd tell you to take every opportunity you can to nurture yourself.

The late Louise Hay said that it is so important that parents love themselves first. She believed if we all did, it would be a much more loving world. We'd be not only caring for our kids differently, we'd be teaching them – modeling for them - self-care and self-love, too.

Let me take some of the guilt away. Caring for yourself is not selfish. It is necessary. Let me also tell the parent who has to keep working not to feel guilty. You can't be everywhere at once. Play your part to the best of your ability.

Probably, the sort of cancer your child has is different from Yousef's. Maybe he or she is older or younger than Yousef was. Maybe different things complicated your life or got in the way of your child's treatment. But many of the same things are true: you must take care of yourself, stay in the present, breathe, look for the beautiful and the positive, and find the love.

It has become so clear to me how much more research is still needed for children's cancer. Here in Sweden, the Childhood Cancer Foundation's goal is to eradicate cancer, but as I see it, it really needs to be a worldwide effort.

I have become very aware of the need for aftercare – support for the family once the child is released from the hospital, told to go home and take the treatments prescribed, and get the child in school again and begin life over. After all the support of round-the-clock nursing care, it is scary to bring home a child and know it's only you now. After being a part of a protocol that tells you exactly what to do if something medical comes up with your child, now we have to explain how he is a cancer survivor to every doctor or dentist we see. Some won't treat him for the most basic things, because now, post-cancer, things are complicated – and maybe they fear doing something wrong. I imagine having to explain the diagnosis and treatment over and over until Yousef is old enough to tell himself whenever he needs a routine booster shot for this or an ordinary prescription for that.

My goal with this book was to give some hope and comfort from my own family's experience. I want you to know there is an end, though you may not see it yet, and I don't know what it is for you. The first thought most parents have is that their child will die. But know that there are so many survivors, more and more every year. So rather than sink in fear, believe your child will be one of the survivors. And to keep doing that, you must do everything in your power to remember that your thoughts are just thoughts.

Bless you and your family as you go through an ordeal you could neither prepare for nor anticipate. Know you are not alone, and may you look for blessings along the way.

## My Notes

# Afterword: Now

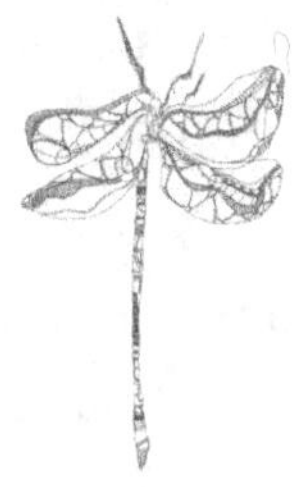

You cannot go back.

But,

Who you are doesn't end.

You are different –

He is different.

"Look how I run!" my 11-year-old starting-over

child calls to me.

Look how he has learned.

To run.

Regardless that he has lived in his body and

learned these things before.

This is your child too. Or will be.

She may have to learn how to speak, how to see,

how to move.

She, like a baby, starts to walk and learn new things – because now she is a different person.

We are a different family.

And so are you.

I cheer on my starting-over child. I watch him run.

You will not be the same.

But you will have so much more.

Than before.

You are not alone.

# Using the Power of Questions

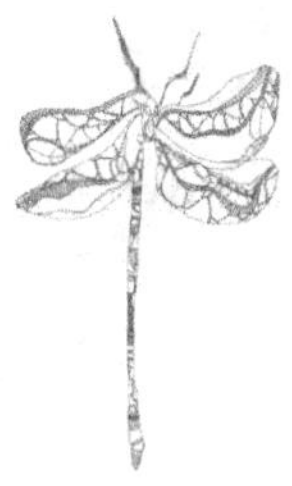

If there is a tough choice, time or place, ask:

What can I do to change this for the greater?

What else is possible here?

What is this?

What can I do with this?

Can I change it?

How do I change it?

If I was to choose what's true for me, what would I be choosing?

What's right about this?

What am I good at that will be easy for me and helpful now?

What awareness do I have here?

What else might I choose to feel right now?